T0208805

CAPNOGRAPHY
King of the ABC's
A Systematic Approach for Paramedics

Troy Valente, BA, Nationally Registered Paramedic
Firefighter/Paramedic in Northern Colorado
Bachelor of Arts in Exercise Science
Sports Medicine Minor

iUniverse, Inc.
New York   Bloomington

Capnography, King of the ABC's
A Systematic Approach for Paramedics

iUniverse books may be ordered through booksellers or by contacting:

iUniverse
1663 Liberty Drive
Bloomington, IN 47403
www.iuniverse.com
1-800-Authors (1-800-288-4677)

ISBN: 978-1-4502-4620-0 (pbk)
ISBN: 978-1-4502-4621-7 (ebk)

Printed in the United States of America

iUniverse rev. date: 7/30/2010

Special Thanks To . . .

My wife, Barbara Valente, RN, BSN, for her incredible support and mad editing skills

Dr. Baruch Krauss, MD, Harvard Medical School & Children's Hospital of Boston, for his mentorship and contributions

Sarah Wooten, DVM, for her friendship and editing input

Rick Smith, Fire Lieutenant/Paramedic, for his friendship, mentorship and contributions

Jeff Stranahan, Fire Lieutenant/Paramedic, for his friendship and mentorship

Mary Mast, RN for her friendship, mentorship and numerous opportunities for growth and development

The incredible men and women in Colorado serving Greeley Fire/Rescue, Pridemark Paramedic Services and Weld County Paramedic Services

PREFACE

My EMS career began in the summer of 2002 as a Firefighter/EMT. Before that, I completed a B.A. in Exercise Science with a Sports Medicine minor: 3 years at Pepperdine University and 1 year at The University of Northern Colorado. In 2006, I attended paramedic school and was turned on to capnography by one of my preceptors during my field internship. Carbon dioxide production and elimination as well as the effects on acid/base balance was something very familiar to me from my studies in exercise physiology and my personal experience as a competitive collegiate endurance athlete. This background was a great segue into capnography and I quickly developed an appetite for more knowledge.

I soon realized that unless I caught a yearly presentation at an EMS conference or the occasional article, there were limited opportunities for learning more about capnography as it relates to paramedicine; no book, nothing. My only option was sifting through blogs and talking to other medics hoping that the information I was getting was accurate. Hence, this book evolved as a diary of my learning process in hopes that other paramedics who wanted to learn about capnography in EMS could do so with better ease in the future.

In July of 2008, Dr. Baruch Krauss agreed to mentor me through the writing process and ensure that I was being accurate in my application of capnography into EMS, particularly when discussing non-intubated applications as the research in this area is very limited. Dr. Baruch Krauss is a nationally renowned capnography researcher and educator who works as an attending physician for Children's Hospital in Boston and is an associate professor of pediatrics for Harvard Medical School. His influence to this text has been invaluable and insured its accuracy.

Capnography texts have been written in the clinical settings of anesthesiology, critical care and ventilator management ad nauseum, but never for the paramedic.....until now. Hopefully, this book will serve as the foundation for all paramedics to develop a full understanding of capnography as it applies to EMS.

TABLE OF CONTENTS

CHAPTER I: THE BASICS

The Greeks seem to get credit for everything and capnography is no exception. They were the first to believe that the body had a central combustion center and that this system had a byproduct. They named this byproduct *Capnos*, which is Greek for "Smoke". Today, we call this combustion center "metabolism" and *Capnos* "carbon dioxide (CO_2)". Simply put, CO_2 is the "smoke" of metabolism[1].

Capnography uses infrared light to measure CO_2 in exhaled air providing accurate and reliable information regarding a patient's airway, breathing and circulation (ABC's) and metabolic status[1]. There are three main capnography technologies used to measure CO_2:

1. <u>Waveform Capnography</u> – displays a waveform with the horizontal axis representing expiration time and the vertical axis representing mmHg of CO_2.
2. <u>Capnometer</u> – measures the patient's peak CO_2 concentration in each breath, called "end tidal carbon dioxide" (ETCO$_2$), and the patient's respiratory rate (RR).
3. <u>Colorimetric Capnography</u> – a device containing litmus paper that changes color when it comes in contact with CO_2.

For the purpose of this text, "capnography" will refer to the simultaneous use of waveform and capnometer technologies as this is the most common configuration used in EMS.

It is important for the paramedic to understand the high reliability and accuracy of capnography. In fact, capnography is considered by many experts to be a diagnostic test[1]. Capnography is also very sensitive, operating at sampling rates as low as 50mL/minute[2]. However, diagnostic tests, regardless of their ability and value, must be interpreted in the context of the patient's clinical picture. For example, in 8th grade I had a severe case of bacterial pneumonia. The infection was so consolidated that the radiologist diagnosed me with lymphoma of the lung as the pneumonia looked like a massive tumor! Yet when our family doctor interpreted the x-ray through the lens of my presentation, it was clear that this was a serious case of pneumonia and not cancer. Therefore, if an x-ray can be misconstrued when interpreted outside of a clinical context, capnography is no exception.

Additionally, be aware that diagnostic tests have technological limits. If my doctor needed more in-depth information on a specific pathology involved with my lung tissue, he would have had to order an MRI due to the limitations of an x-ray. Like an x-ray, capnography has technological limitations, particularly in patients experiencing a simultaneous V/Q mismatch (see chapter II) and certain artifact situations (discussed later in chapter I).

Finally, as with all good tools, improper application and/or prioritization in their use can be counterproductive and/or detrimental. For example, if a patient is in respiratory distress, the first priority should be high flow oxygen, not capnography. Although capnography will often allow the paramedic to be more efficient in reaching a specific differential diagnosis, it is still part of a bigger picture that must be completed; do not abandon other assessments as no diagnostic test is a "tell all".

Throughout this text, paramedics will not only explore the technical side of capnography and its limitations, they will also learn to prioritize, apply and interpret capnography appropriately and routinely in the clinical context of various patients.

Capnography "Tech Talk"

Capnography is able to sample exhaled air through two different technologies: side-stream and main-stream. Side-Stream Capnography samples and then analyzes the patient's exhaled air "off to the side" away from the patient's direct path of exhalation. Main-Stream Capnography places the CO_2 analyzer in the patient's direct path of exhalation. Side-stream is a newer technology that has replaced most main-stream devices and is the most common technology used in EMS. Neonatal capnography may still benefit from main-stream technology due to the low tidal volumes of neonatal patients. However, side-stream capnography is still used in neonate patients depending on the clinical situation[3].

There are two types of waveform capnography: time and volumetric. In time capnography, CO_2 is measured over time and in volumetric capnography CO_2 is measured over tidal volume. Time capnography is used in the pre-hospital setting as volumetric capnography requires equipment that is too cumbersome for EMS. However, volumetric capnography can be very useful in certain disease processes, particularly when dealing with alveolar dead space and/or extremely low tidal volumes, allowing clinicians to further investigate the initial findings of time capnography[4].

Capnography vs. Pulse Oximetry

While capnography and pulse oximetry may seem like similar measurements, they actually assess very different things. Capnography is a measurement of ventilation and, indirectly, circulatory and metabolic status. Pulse oximetry measures the color of the hemoglobin (Hgb) molecule and then uses mathematic algorithms to estimate the percent of Hgb saturation.

Hemoglobin is a helix-type molecule that coils tighter and appears redder the more saturated it becomes; it uncoils and appears bluer the less saturated it is. The redder/bluer the Hgb the higher/lower the saturation percentage estimated by pulse oximetry. An important technological limitation of pulse oximetry is that it cannot decipher what is bound to the Hgb molecule. This becomes crucial to understand in the context of carbon monoxide poisoning.

Carbon monoxide is 200 times more attracted to hemoglobin than oxygen. Therefore, a patient with carbon monoxide poisoning will read 100% on their pulse oximetry as carbon monoxide's higher affinity causes the Hbg molecule to coil tightly and appear very red (hence the textbook "cherry red" appearance of postmortem carbon monoxide patients). However, a patient with carbon monoxide poisoning is hypoxemic and NOT oxygenated.

Other issues arise with pulse oximetry as well. There are significant delays in measuring pulse oximetry in the finger from what is going on centrally in the core. This is the biggest reason for central pulse oximetry monitoring on critical patients, particularly pediatric patients. If a patient becomes apneic, it could take up to several minutes for the patient's pulse oximetry to change. In fact, I once had an anesthesiologist tell me that a healthy adult can maintain their oxygen saturation for up to 10 minutes without breathing! On the other hand, capnography instantly detects that a patient has stopped breathing.

Additional problems with pulse oximetry are related to intermittent readings, usually secondary to artifact caused by low perfusion, cold fingers, fingernail polish, long finger nails, patient movement, your partner hits a curb at 90 mph, etc. Nonetheless, pulse oximetry still has its value as long as the paramedic interprets and uses pulse oximetry in the context of its technological limitations and uses it in conjunction with capnography to complete the clinical picture.

Carbon Dioxide (CO_2) Unveiled

CO_2 is produced after bicarbonate buffers the acidic byproducts of metabolism and is then transported by the blood to the lungs where it diffuses across the alveolar membrane and is exhaled. The diffusion rate of CO_2 is 20 times faster than that of oxygen (O_2) due to its higher solubility[5]. This is an important concept to grasp when discussing the capnography of congestive heart failure (CHF) (see chapter III) as this high solubility allows CO_2 to diffuse at the same rate through fluid as it does through air[1]. 60% of CO_2 is carried by the bicarbonate buffering system, 30% is typically bound to hemoglobin, and the other 10% is dissolved in plasma, the watery portion of the blood[5]. Below is an oversimplified equation illustrating CO_2 production (may the chemistry gods forgive me). The equation is reversible and can move left to right (increasing pH) or right to left (decreasing pH) in order to maintain a homeostatic acid/base balance.

$$\text{Acid } (H^+) + \text{Bicarbonate } (HCO_3^-) <=> CO_2 + H_2O$$

For the sake of conceptual learning and at the expense of chemistry, think of CO_2 as an acid in gas form. The body is constantly eliminating acid by converting it to CO_2, allowing it to be exhaled. During hypoventilation CO_2 builds up in the blood decreasing pH (respiratory acidosis). During hyperventilation the rate of CO_2 elimination is too high, increasing pH (respiratory alkalosis). Furthermore, if hypoventilation or hyperventilation persists long enough and/or a metabolic issue ensues that overwhelms the respiratory system, the renal system will have to manipulate bicarbonate levels in order to maintain a homeostatic pH (metabolic acidosis/alkalosis). While only blood gas analysis can quantitatively determine if a patient is in respiratory or metabolic acidosis or alkalosis, capnography can give qualitative insight into these conditions through a V/Q assessment (see chapter II).

$ETCO_2$ vs. $PaCO_2$

End tidal carbon dioxide ($ETCO_2$) is the technical term for the amount of CO_2 measured in expired air via capnography. The actual unit of $ETCO_2$ is a measurement of pressure reported in millimeters of mercury (mmHg). $ETCO_2$ is normally 35-45 mmHg in a healthy individual[2]. Several factors can change a person's $ETCO_2$, such as RR and their circulatory/metabolic status (these will be discussed later on).

During respiratory distress, ventilations become ineffective leading to decreased gas exchange, hypercapnia and a rise in $ETCO_2$. While a rise in $ETCO_2$ does not directly cause respiratory failure, it is an indicator to the severity of the respiratory issue. There is no definite $ETCO_2$ value that indicates when respiratory distress has become severe enough to cause respiratory failure, as it depends on the patient's baseline $ETCO_2$ levels and the respiratory pathology involved. However, research indicates that in patients with normal $ETCO_2$ values for their baseline, an $ETCO_2$ of approximately 70-80 mmHg[6] is a reliable indicator that their respiratory distress is severe enough for respiratory failure to be eminent. Some patients could experience respiratory failure with higher/lower $ETCO_2$ levels depending on the pathology of their disease and the corresponding effects on baseline $ETCO_2$ levels.

Partial pressure of arterial carbon dioxide ($PaCO_2$) is the measurement of CO_2 pressure in arterial blood that is obtained through lab values. In healthy patients, $ETCO_2$ and $PaCO_2$ can be used interchangeably as they only vary by 1-5 mmHg[7] or 2%-7%[8]. During disease, the difference between $PaCO_2$ and $ETCO_2$, called the "$PaCO_2$ - $ETCO_2$ gradient", can indicate the severity of the pathology[6].

Physiologic Waveforms

As discussed earlier, capnography can provide more than just numbers; it can display a waveform as well. There are two waveform groups: physiologic and artifact. Physiologic waveforms are related to patient physiology and can be diagnostic while artifact waveforms are neither. Following are several physiologic waveforms that paramedics could possibly see in the field, including an explanation of their origin. Note that the waveforms included are not an exhaustive list but rather the most pertinent to paramedicine.

A normal capnography waveform in a healthy individual looks like a plateau with fairly vertical sides and has four phases[1,2]:

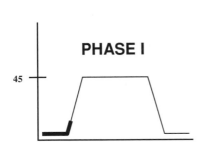

Phase I represents the exhalation of "dead air", or air that does not reach the alveoli for gas exchange. Dead air fills the upper airway and upper portions of the lower airway and contains no CO_2. Phase I ends with the initial detection of CO_2.

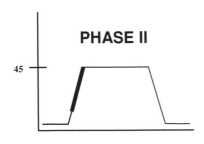

Phase II represents alveolar air, rich in CO_2 from gas exchange, as it initially reaches the upper airway and is detected causing a sharp rise in the waveform.

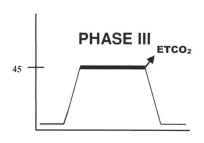

Phase III represents CO_2 being evenly distributed from the alveoli to the upper airway. The slope of phase III is very important in determining any delays in the exhalation of alveolar air and the severity of such delays. The end of phase III, the highest point, is the peak CO_2 concentration and is where the capnometer provides a number for the patient's $ETCO_2$.

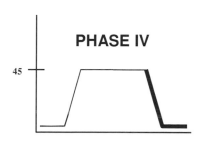

Phase IV represents inhalation. $ETCO_2$ levels quickly fall to zero as atmospheric air is measured during inhalation, which does not contain enough CO_2 to be detected by capnography (my apologies to the greenhouse gas committee).

Below is a capnogram of a normal waveform. You should be comfortable identifying and physiologically describing all the phases before moving on:

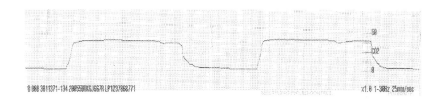

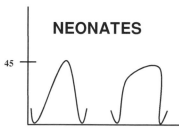

Neonates often have an exaggerated phase II and a shortened or missing phase III. This is due to lower tidal volumes, increased respiratory rates and smaller airways[3]. However, $ETCO_2$ values are the same for all healthy individuals. Normal lung function is normal lung function regardless of age[1].

The Proverbial "Shark Fin"

During bronchial constriction, it takes longer for air to be exhaled from the lungs. This increase in expiratory time causes phase II and III to slur and eventually merge together, creating a "shark fin" appearance. A shark fin waveform is as diagnostic to bronchial constriction as ST elevation is to an MI. Additionally, the more phase II and III slur together and/or the steeper the slope to phase III, the more severe the bronchial constriction pathology. Note that some individuals naturally have a slight slope to phase III[1,2].

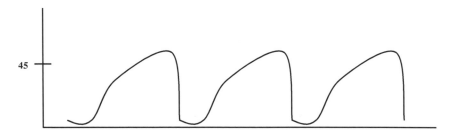

Hyperventilation

During hyperventilation the waveform narrows as a result of a decreased expiratory time (increased respiratory rate) and shortens due to decreased $ETCO_2$ as a result of decreasing $PaCO_2$ (hypocapnia). In other words, CO_2 is eliminated more quickly than it is delivered to the lungs[9].

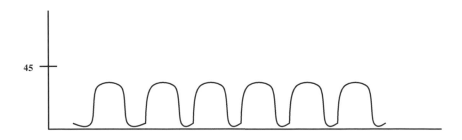

Classic Hypoventilation

During classic hypoventilation, technically called "bradypneic hypoventilation", the waveform widens as a result of an increased expiratory time (decreased respiratory rate) and grows taller due to increased $ETCO_2$ as a result of climbing $PaCO_2$ (hypercapnia). In other words, CO_2 is delivered to the lungs more quickly than it is eliminated. Classic hypoventilation occurs in the presence of normal tidal volumes and is commonly seen in opioid overdoses[1, 6].

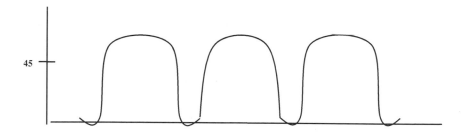

Atypical Hypoventilation

Atypical hypoventilation, technically called "hypopneic hypoventilation", occurs most commonly in procedural sedation, analgesia and seizures. This counterintuitive phenomenon causes normal or decreased $ETCO_2$ despite a low RR and hypercapnia. Atypical hypoventilation occurs when tidal volume becomes excessively lower than the patient's already low RR. Even though CO_2 is still being delivered to the lungs faster than it is being exhaled and $PaCO_2$ is increasing (hypercapnia), the patient's low tidal volume creates a decreased capacity for gas exchange. Depending on the severity of the patient's low tidal volume, $ETCO_2$ may be normal or low, but it will not be high like it is in classic hypoventilation where tidal volumes are adequate. Note that further assessments are required to distinguish a low $ETCO_2$ caused by atypical hypoventilation vs. a circulatory or metabolic issue (see V/Q discussions in chapter II)[1, 6].

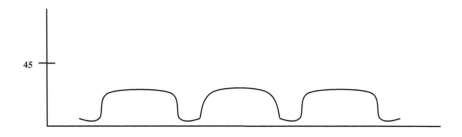

Apnea Etiology Differentiation

Apnea can be detected by capnography almost instantaneously and is represented by a flat line similar to asystole on the electrocardiogram (ECG).

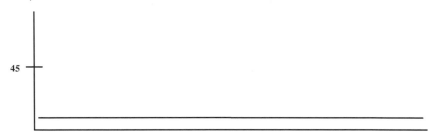

There are two types of apnea: obstructive and central. Obstructive apnea, such as during complete laryngeal spasm or choking, can be diagnosed by chest wall movement in the presence of a flat line capnogram. Central apnea is depicted by a flat line with no chest wall movement.

Partial airway obstructions from food or objects can be distinguished from partial laryngeal spasm based on the response to interventions. Often, partial airway obstruction will resolve through airway alignment/positioning. However, partial laryngeal spasms do not respond to these techniques[1,6].

Phase III Upswing

In obese or pregnant patients that are being ventilated, or less commonly spontaneously breathing, decreased thoracic compliance may alter alveolar emptying resulting in a late upswing to phase III[10]. This waveform abnormality may occur intermittently or continuously. Ensure that the patient's ventilatory status is effective and/or assist them into a lateral recumbent position. If seen in a patient who is not obese or pregnant, consider an artifact origin (see Artifact Waveforms).

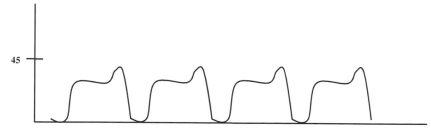

Rebreathing

While managing a patient who is intubated, on a non-rebreather mask (NRBM) or on continuous positive airway pressure (CPAP), CO_2 can re-enter the patient's breathing circuit causing a steady rise in the waveform baseline. Rebreathing is more common in patients under anesthesia or on ventilators but possible for paramedics to see in the field, particularly with CPAP treatments. If observed, ensure that the breathing circuit or CPAP mask is void of equipment malfunctions[9].

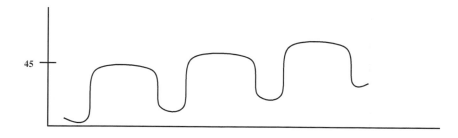

Curare Cleft

A dip in phase III, called a curare cleft, is caused by diaphragm movement in the absence of thoracic muscle movement. This waveform may be seen when an intubated patient spontaneously breathes on their own, during CPR, in certain spinal injuries and other circumstances that would cause isolated diaphragm movement[11]. In spontaneously breathing patients a curare cleft is most likely caused by artifact.

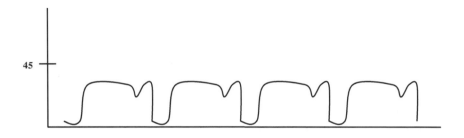

Cardiac Oscillations

Cardiac oscillations are caused by the heart as it beats against the lungs and can only be seen during ineffective breathing patterns associated with either profound hypoventilation and/or small tidal volumes. While this phenomenon is rare, it is always indicative of ineffective breathing and a life threatening situation[11].

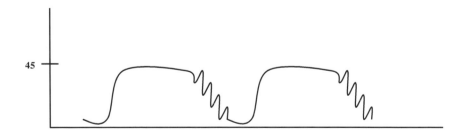

Artifact Waveforms

In contrast to physiologic waveforms, artifact waveforms are caused by factors that are not necessarily a direct result of patient physiology. Simply put, if the paramedic cannot confidently equate the waveform to a physiologic origin, consider an artifact cause. IMPORTANT: Always rule out life threatening causes of abnormal waveforms prior to assuming the waveform is caused by artifact, particularly in patients with altered mentation and/or patients who have been intubated. Do not confuse artifact waveforms with ineffective breathing, a tube that has migrated into the hypopharynx and/or a tube cuff that is leaking. Nonetheless, it is important for paramedics to be aware of artifact waveforms to avoid a "physiological goose chase" for a cause that may simply be artifact. Know that the occasional artifact waveform is very common. However, the presence of continuous artifact waveforms indicates that $ETCO_2$ and RR values are possibly unreliable. To the contrary, the absence of artifact waveforms ensures that the capnography equipment is working properly. Examples of artifact waveforms are shown below:

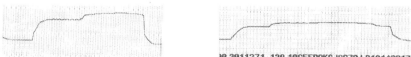

Stair-stepping waveforms with a constant baseline (not to be confused with rebreathing that has a rising baseline)

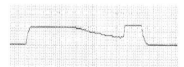

Poly-shaped waveforms

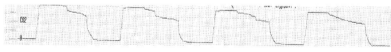

Negatively sloped waveforms

Listed below are some common causes of artifact waveforms:

- <u>Talking</u> – While movement is not an issue with capnography like it is with an ECG, expiratory patterns change during speech causing random waveform shapes.
- <u>High Flow Oxygen</u> – Oxygen treatments, such as a NRBM or CPAP, sometimes cause sampling flow interference due to the turbulent environment inside the mask.
- <u>Gunk 'N Junk</u> – Bodily secretions blocking flow in and out of the tube and/or sampler can change the waveform shape or cause the capnography to quit working altogether if the sensor becomes completely clogged.
- <u>Excessive Mouth Breathing</u> – Encourage patients to breath in and out of their nose in order to eliminate artifact waveforms.
- <u>Fiddling</u> – Patients sometimes play with the upper lip cannula piece which can change the waveform shape.
- <u>Unique Anatomical Characteristics</u> – Not all patients read the textbook. Sometimes they have unexplained capnography that is normal to their physiology. Use good judgment, particularly with intubated patients, as an abnormal waveform can indicate a problem with tube placement and/or airway patency.

Hopefully the concepts presented in this chapter have established some basic knowledge for the paramedic to build on throughout the next few chapters as the text dives deeper into the type of feedback capnography can provide and how to interpret such findings. If you are very new to capnography, it is recommended that you put yourself on capnography and try to become familiar with finding and interpreting these basic concepts before moving further through the text.

References

1. B. Krauss (personal communication, 2008 through 2009).
2. Krauss, B, Silvestri, S, and Falk, J. (2008). Carbon dioxide monitoring (capnography). Retrieved October 18, 2008 from www.uptodate.com.
3. Schmalisch, G. Time and Volumetric Capnography in the Neonates. In Gravenstein, J.S., Jaffee, M.B. and Paulus, D.A. (Ed.), *Capnography: Clinical Aspects* (81 – 99). 2004. Cambridge, U.K.: Cambridge University Press.
4. Gravenstein, J.S., Paulus, D.A. Clinical Perspectives. In Gravenstein, J.S., Jaffee, M.B. and Paulus, D.A. (Ed.), *Capnography: Clinical Aspects* (3 – 12). 2004. Cambridge, U.K.: Cambridge University Press.
5. West, J.B. *Pulmonary Physiology and Pathophysiology: An Integrated, Case-Based Approach* (2nd Ed.) (6, 12). 2007. Baltimore, MD: Lippincott Williams & Wilkins.
6. Krauss, B and Hess, D. Capnography for Procedural Sedation and Analgesia in the Emergency Department. *Annals of Emergency Medicine,* 2007, 50: 172-181.
7. Lobato, E.B., Kirby, R.R. Capnography and Respiratory Assessment Outside of the Operating Room. In Gravenstein, J.S., Jaffee, M.B. and Paulus, D.A. (Ed.), *Capnography: Clinical Aspects* (15 – 20). 2004. Cambridge, U.K.: Cambridge University Press.
8. Greenway, L. Non-Invasive End-Tidal Carbon Dioxide Monitoring in Conjunction with Non-Invasive Positive Pressure Ventilation. In Gravenstein, J.S., Jaffee, M.B. and Paulus, D.A. (Ed.), *Capnography: Clinical Aspects* (137 – 142). 2004. Cambridge, U.K.: Cambridge University Press.
9. Unknown Author(s). Appendix: Patterns of Time-Based Capnograms. In Gravenstein, J.S., Jaffee, M.B. and Paulus, D.A. (Ed.), *Capnography: Clinical Aspects* (427 – 431). 2004. Cambridge, U.K.: Cambridge University Press.
10. Kodali, B. (2008). *Capnography: A Comprehensive Educational Website.* Retrieved July 2009 from www.capnography.com.
11. Smalhout, B. The First Years of Clinical Capnography. In Gravenstein, J.S., Jaffee, M.B. and Paulus, D.A. (Ed.), *Capnography: Clinical Aspects* (355 – 379). 2004. Cambridge, U.K.: Cambridge University Press

CHAPTER II:
A SYSTEMATIC APPROACH

Several considerations were given to writing this text:
1. Paramedics needed a comprehensive source for information on using and interpreting capnography in the context of the pre-hospital environment.
2. There was no text addressing the use and interpretation of capnography on spontaneously breathing patients, the most common application in EMS.
3. Paramedics also needed a simple, systematic approach for using capnography.

Hence, the text before you evolved as a diary of the author's learning process with chapters II and III at its heart. Throughout this chapter the paramedic will develop a systematic approach to use in the field. Additionally, the paramedic will learn how to qualitatively determine a patient's V/Q ratio from their capnography. Remember, that while capnography has enormous value, it should not be prioritized above urgent BLS interventions. For example, do not delay high flow oxygen therapy in critical respiratory patients just to get an initial capnography reading.

The Initial Impression

It is important to use capnography frequently at first, particularly for newer medics or medics unfamiliar with capnography, in order to develop an approach that becomes second nature and unique to your style of medicine. Of course, any approach can be modified as needed. However, if a systematic approach is not developed, the paramedic will have a difficult time feeling comfortable using capnography in critical circumstances that require faster progression and/or a quicker thought process. Therefore, capnography should be used as much as possible initially. As the paramedic becomes more comfortable, he/she can decrease capnography use to patients with ABC and/or mentation issues as well any patient that has the potential to deteriorate. When using capnography, paramedics can adopt the following simple, three-step systematic approach for incorporating and interpreting capnography in their medicine:

1. Initial Impression (a.k.a. "The Doorway Diagnosis") paying close attention to patient color, mentation and respiratory effort.
2. Categorical Waveform Analysis.
3. Qualitative V/Q ratio analysis derived from the $ETCO_2$/RR relationship.

The doorway diagnosis begins to paint the necessary clinical picture within which capnography will be interpreted. This initial impression occurs on approach to the patient and pays close attention to the patient's respiratory effort, color and mentation. These three observations are specifically chosen as they stand alone in answering the proverbial question "sick or not sick"? For example, tachypnea by itself is not automatically indicative of a sick patient from an initial impression perspective. However, tachypnea associated with increased respiratory effort, a color change and/or decreased mentation is immediately concerning. An initial impression is dynamic and does not stop at the doorway, but changes and flexes as more information is gained in the subsequent patient assessments.

Placing capnography in the patient's clinical picture is critical for accurate interpretation. For example, some patients have higher than normal $ETCO_2$ levels unrelated to COPD pathologies and/or a slight slope to phase III. If these patients' capnography is interpreted outside of their clinical picture, the paramedic's differential diagnosis and treatment plan will be grossly inaccurate. They are not sick; their physiology is just out of the norm. A good initial impression will make or break how smoothly and/or effectively a paramedic runs a call.

Waveform Analysis

Once a working doorway diagnosis indicates the need for capnography, rule out the need for immediate BLS interventions, such as high flow oxygen. Then, apply capnography and observe the waveform in the context of your initial impression. Decipher whether the waveform is physiologic or artifact. If the waveform is physiologic, decide what is categorically revealed about the patient. If the waveform is artifact, begin to rule out causes of artifact waveforms.

Systematic Capnography

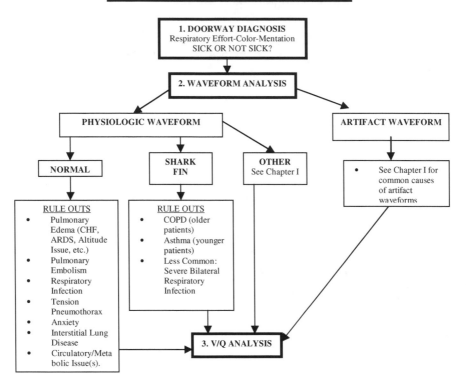

1. DOORWAY DIAGNOSIS
Respiratory Effort-Color-Mentation
SICK OR NOT SICK?

2. WAVEFORM ANALYSIS

PHYSIOLOGIC WAVEFORM

ARTIFACT WAVEFORM

NORMAL

SHARK FIN

OTHER
See Chapter I

- See Chapter I for common causes of artifact waveforms

RULE OUTS
- Pulmonary Edema (CHF, ARDS, Altitude Issue, etc.)
- Pulmonary Embolism
- Respiratory Infection
- Tension Pneumothorax
- Anxiety
- Interstitial Lung Disease
- Circulatory/Metabolic Issue(s).

RULE OUTS
- COPD (older patients)
- Asthma (younger patients)
- Less Common: Severe Bilateral Respiratory Infection

3. V/Q ANALYSIS

The V/Q Ratio

Once the paramedic has completed the initial impression, provided BLS interventions of an immediate nature and assessed the waveform, the third step involves analyzing the patient's V/Q ratio. An understanding of the V/Q ratio is the "gold nugget" of capnography as it can give the deepest insight into the patient's physiology. However, in order to grasp the V/Q ratio concept, the paramedic must first have a complete understanding of what governs RR and how respiratory, circulatory and metabolic changes affect $ETCO_2$ values.

For the healthy individual, respiratory rate (RR) is governed by the partial pressure of CO_2 (pCO_2) as monitored by the medulla centers of the brainstem with a "back-up" system in the hypothalamus monitoring pH[1]. As these respiratory centers sense a rise in pCO_2, they signal the respiratory muscles to increase the rate of breathing. By increasing RR, a person is able to blow off excess CO_2, returning the pCO_2 to normal. If a healthy individual hyperventilates, pCO_2 decreases (hypocapnia) causing their $ETCO_2$ to drop below normal as more CO_2 is being blown off than is being delivered to the lungs. To the contrary, if a healthy individual hypoventilates pCO_2 builds up in the blood resulting in higher than normal $ETCO_2$ levels (hypercapnia) as more CO_2 is delivered to the lungs than is being blown off.

Hypocapnia   Hypercapnia

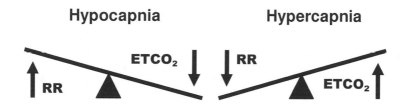

In patients with chronic CO_2 retention, the body becomes desensitized to high pCO_2 levels much like the body becomes desensitized to chronically high blood glucose levels and the associated insulin response in Type II Diabetes. Consequently, the body begins to monitor the partial pressure of oxygen (pO_2) instead of pCO_2 dictating RR based on changes in pO_2; this is referred to as a "hypoxic drive".

The effect that the respiratory system can have on $ETCO_2$ levels is well illustrated by the CO_2 retention often seen in respiratory pathologies. While not all respiratory patients retain CO_2, patients that do usually have 1, 2 or all 3 of the following etiologies at work:

1. Chronic Obstructive Pulmonary Disease (COPD) – typically involves the classic marriage between emphysema and chronic bronchitis caused by years of smoking and/or environmental exposure(s). Although, research has found a genetic link to emphysema (alpha-1 antitrypsin deficiency) explaining why some patients develop emphysema without ever having been exposed to the typical risk factors[7]. Delayed alveolar diffusion rates caused by emphysema, and exhalation delays caused by chronic bronchitis from mutated mucous centers producing increased mucous, all explain why this type of patient typically suffers from chronic CO_2 retention.

2. Asthma – may be chronic or acute. Chronic bronchial constriction and the corresponding mucous production from inflammation results in chronic CO_2 retention. Depending on the severity of an acute asthma attack, CO_2 retention may or may not occur. The capnography of acute asthma attacks as well as an explanation on why asthma and COPD are being presented as separate etiologies will be further discussed in chapter III.

3. Ineffective Ventilations – the causes of ineffective ventilations are numerous. Nonetheless, when this etiology is present gas exchange is impaired leading to hypercapnia and high $ETCO_2$ values.

To understand the capnography of CO_2 retention, the paramedic needs to understand that $ETCO_2$ is a measurement of pressure and is directly affected by the pCO_2 in the pulmonary circulation. Regardless of whether the etiology is chronic or acute, when a patient retains CO_2, a "bottleneck traffic jam" ensues in the pulmonary circulation causing "back pressure", which results in hypercapnia and increases in $ETCO_2$. CO_2 retaining patients compensate for their condition by having a higher than normal RR to combat their hypercapnia (as well as their hypoxia) and may also retain bicarbonate to combat metabolic acidosis if the pathology is chronic.

In addition to the respiratory system, the patient's circulatory and metabolic status can affect $ETCO_2$ as well. The CO_2 Circuit describes the relationships between all of the circulatory and metabolic components, as well as respiratory factors, that can affect $ETCO_2$:

- Oxygen, Nutrients & Perfusion – All are necessary for normal metabolic activity. For example, if a patient is hypovolemic, experiencing a cardiac event, hypoxic and/or emaciated, metabolic activity decreases leading to less CO_2 production and lower $ETCO_2$ levels.
- Metabolism – Anything that affects metabolic activity levels will affect CO_2 production and $ETCO_2$ levels. For instance, if a patient is experiencing a thyroid storm, fever or malignant hyperthermia, metabolic activity increases resulting in increased CO_2 production equating to a higher $ETCO_2$.

- <u>CO_2 Production</u> - CO_2 production is not only dependent on metabolic activity levels, but also adequate bicarbonate levels to be able to buffer acid. For example, if a patient is in diabetic ketoacidosis or cardiac arrest, bicarbonate levels can be depleted resulting in dramatically low CO_2 production and $ETCO_2$ levels (metabolic acidosis). Or, excess bicarbonate levels can result in increased acid buffering (metabolic alkalosis) increasing CO_2 production and $ETCO_2$ levels.
- <u>Delivery & Exhalation</u> – This component of the CO_2 circuit includes the respiratory etiologies previously discussed. Anything affecting the delivery, diffusion across the alveolar membrane and exhalation of CO_2, such as COPD or a pulmonary embolism (PE), will affect $ETCO_2$ levels.

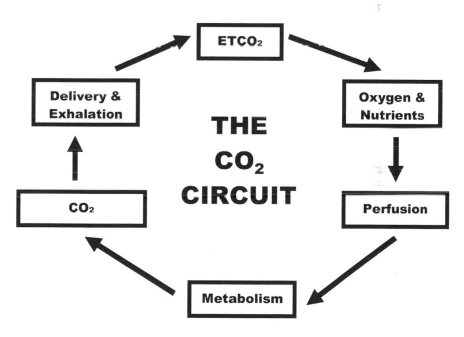

A change anywhere in the CO_2 circuit has the potential to affect $ETCO_2$ levels. By understanding the complete picture of respiratory, circulatory and metabolic factors that have the potential to affect $ETCO_2$ levels, the paramedic can better understand and utilize the V/Q assessment capabilities of capnography.

The V/Q ratio compares the volume of air being ventilated in the lungs (V) with the amount of blood being delivered to the lungs (Q):

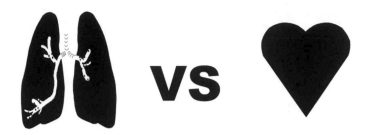

A normal V/Q ratio is 0.8 with 4L of air being ventilated per minute for every 5L of blood delivered (4/5 = 0.8). A V/Q mismatch occurs when the delicate "tug-of-war" between ventilation and pulmonary perfusion "seesaws" out of balance. If RR increases and/or pulmonary perfusion decreases a V/Q mismatch of >.8 occurs. For example, if a patient begins hyperventilating 5 liters of air per minute and pulmonary perfusion stays the same, the V/Q ratio climbs: 5/5 = 1. To the contrary, if RR decreases and/or pulmonary perfusion increases a V/Q mismatch of <.8 occurs. For instance, if an overdose patient begins to hypoventilate at 3 liters of air per minute, the V/Q ratio drops: 3/5 = .6. The assessment of the patient's ventilatory and perfusion status determines the fraction; the decimal number is simply a function of changing a fraction to a decimal.

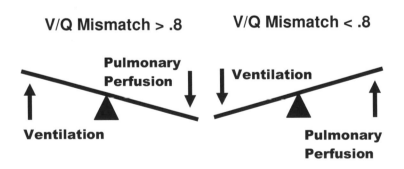

For further illustration, different V/Q ratios are seen in various portions of the lungs themselves without any disease processes. Due to the weight of the lungs, gravity and their vertical orientation, the upper portion of the lungs are better ventilated and less perfused with a V/Q ratio mismatch > 0.8 and the lower portion of the lungs are less ventilated and more perfused with a V/Q ratio mismatch < 0.8[3]:

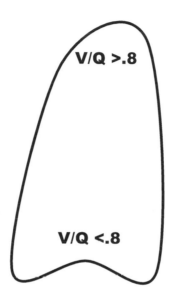

In Capnography, "V" is synonymous with the patient's RR and "Q" is indirectly represented by the patient's $ETCO_2$. While a V/Q ratio assessment traditionally gives a numeric value, capnography is unable to provide a quantitative measurement. Actual values were used here for the sake of learning the V/Q ratio concept. However, capnography can provide *qualitative* information on the V/Q ratio, or mismatch, by placing it into one of 4 categories:

1. <u>Normal V/Q Ratio</u> – Normal $ETCO_2$ and RR values indicate a normal pH.

Normal V/Q Ratio

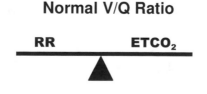

2. <u>Respiratory V/Q Mismatch</u> – Changes in $ETCO_2$ secondary to hyper-/hypoventilation causes a respiratory V/Q mismatch. Low $ETCO_2$ levels explained by hyperventilation indicate respiratory alkalosis, such as seen in anxiety. Likewise, high $ETCO_2$ levels explained by hypoventilation indicate respiratory acidosis, such as seen in an opioid overdose. Remember that atypical hypoventilation also causes respiratory acidosis, although it presents differently, with low $ETCO_2$ secondary to proportionally low tidal volumes and most commonly occurs during procedural sedation, analgesia and seizures (see chapter I).

Hyperventilation
V/Q Mismatch

Hypoventilation
V/Q Mismatch

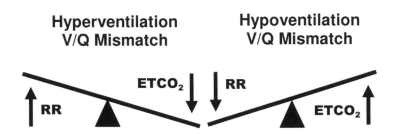

3. <u>Circulatory/Metabolic V/Q Mismatch</u> – ASSUMING A NORMAL RR AND RESPIRATORY STATUS, changes in $ETCO_2$ levels indicate a possible circulatory and/or metabolic issue. Research has shown that an $ETCO_2 > 20$ usually indicates that perfusion is adequate, assuming the patient had normal $ETCO_2$ values to begin with[4]. However, a patient with an $ETCO_2$ in the low to mid 20's that is not explained by RR or a metabolic issue still potentially has a circulatory issue. For example, consider the following vitals of a trauma patient: BP 100/70, 130HR, 20RR, $ETCO_2$ of 22. Obviously, this patient is in compensated shock. Therefore, while an $ETCO_2 > 20$ indicates proper profusion, there could still be a circulatory issue that the body is compensating for. Always complete the full clinical picture with other assessments[6].

Circulatory/Metabolic
V/Q Mismatch

Circulatory/Metabolic
V/Q Mismatch

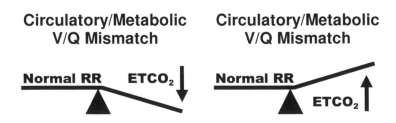

$ETCO_2$ fluctuations from a metabolic issue are caused by bicarbonate level changes and their effect on CO_2 production. Research on pediatric diabetics has found that a threshold $ETCO_2$ of 30 can be used to differentiate a diabetic suffering from high blood sugar who is in metabolic acidosis secondary to DKA (<30 $ETCO_2$), from a diabetic who is not (>30 $ETCO_2$) [4]. This threshold is just a "ballpark" for the paramedic and is only applicable if the diabetic emergency is caught early, prior to the onset of mental status changes and/or Kussmals respirations.

Although rare, metabolic alkalosis secondary to increased bicarbonate levels can explain high $ETCO_2$ levels. ALWAYS, ALWAYS, ALWAYS rule out a respiratory issue first in patients with high $ETCO_2$ levels. Nonetheless, metabolic alkalosis is a real phenomenon and may be caused by prolonged vomiting, renal complications and increased metabolism as seen in fever, hyperthyroid problems, hyperadrenergic states and malignant hyperthermia.

4. <u>Simultaneous V/Q Mismatch</u> – Many disease pathologies have a circulatory, respiratory and/or metabolic component that simultaneously contribute to changes in $ETCO_2$ levels. For example, a patient with a pulmonary embolism (PE) will be hyperventilating to compensate for hypoxia, thus decreasing $ETCO_2$, but will also have compromised pulmonary perfusion, further decreasing $ETCO_2$. Another example is seen in Diabetic Ketoacidosis (DKA). During DKA, prolonged metabolic acidosis depletes bicarbonate levels, which lowers $ETCO_2$. Additionally, Kussmal's respirations develop which also drops $ETCO_2$. Capnography is unable to distinguish between the respiratory, circulatory and/or metabolic contributions to changes in $ETCO_2$ levels in cases where they are simultaneous culprits [5]. As a result, there is an art form involved in order to identify and interpret a simultaneous V/Q mismatch. There are 3 keys to becoming proficient at the art of capnography and being able to interpret a simultaneous V/Q mismatch: complete a full clinical picture of the patient using all assessment tools available, always interpret capnography in the patient's full clinical picture and learn to identify *excessively* low/high $ETCO_2$ levels.

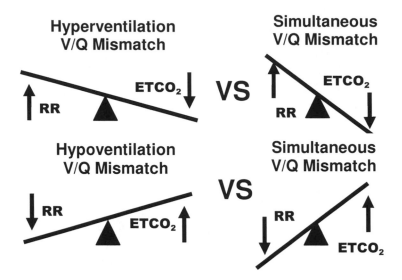

If the $ETCO_2$ level seems too low/high to be explained by RR alone, the paramedic should have a high index of suspicion for a compounding circulatory/metabolic issue depending on the patient's clinical picture. Like any art form, there is no substitute for practice. By continually evaluating V/Q ratios on numerous patients, the paramedic will begin to develop ballpark expectations on $ETCO_2$ levels for patients with various respiratory rates and with different circulatory and/or metabolic pathologies.

While the V/Q assessment is the last step in using capnography systematically and often the most difficult concept to grasp, it is perhaps the most crucial step to learn in order to use capnography to its fullest potential. Chapter III will discuss several etiologies as well as actual cases that illustrate many ways capnography can be used and interpreted in non-intubated patients.

References

1. Schmalisch, G. Respiration at High- and Low-Pressure Environments. In Gravenstein, J.S., Jaffee, M.B. and Paulus, D.A. (Ed.), *Capnography: Clinical Aspects* (121 – 128). 2004. Cambridge, U.K.: Cambridge University Press.

2. West, J.B. *Pulmonary Physiology and Pathophysiology: An Integrated, Case-Based Approach* (2nd Ed.) (31 – 50). 2007. Baltimore, MD: Lippincott Williams & Wilkins.

3. West, J.B. *Pulmonary Physiology and Pathophysiology: An Integrated, Case-Based Approach* (2nd Ed.) (45). 2007. Baltimore, MD: Lippincott Williams & Wilkins.

4. Krauss, B. Advances in the Use of Capnography for Nonintubated Patients. *Israeli Journal of Emergency Medicine*, 2008, 8: 3-15.

5. Krauss, B, Silvestri, S, and Falk, J. (2008). Carbon dioxide monitoring (capnography). Retrieved October 18, 2008 from www.uptodate.com.

6. B. Krauss (personal communication, 2008 through 2009).

7. National Institute of Health (2009). Alpha-1 Antitrypsin Deficiency. Retrieved September 3, 2009 from http://ghr.nlm.nih.gov/condition/alpha-1-antitrypsin-deficiency.

Chapter III: Non-Intubated Applications

Paramedics most often use capnography on spontaneously breathing, non-intubated patients via a nasal cannula. Ironically, references on this application for paramedics to explore the topic further are virtually non-existent. Therefore, this chapter will attempt to give the paramedic a broader understanding of using capnography in non-intubated patients using nasal cannula technologies.

Trending

Trending gives continual feedback on whether the patient is improving or worsening. In respiratory patients, a decrease in $ETCO_2$ levels shows a trend for improvement as ventilations become more effective at gas exchange. If the respiratory patient was worsening, the paramedic would see an increase in $ETCO_2$. Additionally, if a shark fin waveform is present, the paramedic can trend the slope of phase III; less of a slope indicates improvement and a steeper slope indicates a trend for the worse.

Consider the following strip of a 75 yoa female with a COPD exacerbation presenting with 1-3 word dyspnea. Her initial capnography is the top strip (54-64 $ETCO_2$) and her capnography post treatment (Albuterol X 3, 125 mg Solumedrol and 200mL of fluid) is the bottom strip. Not only did her $ETCO_2$ decrease after treatment, the slope of phase III lessened as well. This is an example of trending capnography throughout treatment to obtain objective data indicating that the patient's condition has improved.

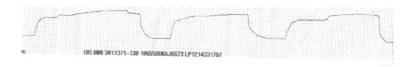

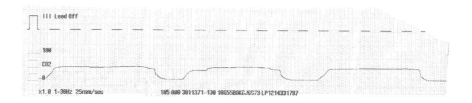

For circulatory/metabolic issues, the paramedic wants to see the $ETCO_2$ trend in the opposite direction of respiratory emergencies. If a patient's circulatory/metabolic situation was improving, we would expect to see the patient's $ETCO_2$ trend higher as the circulatory/metabolic system improves and lower if the patient was worsening. For example, a patient with a severe tension pneumothorax that is compressing the heart and causing a cardiac tamponade will most likely suffer from low $ETCO_2$ levels despite aggressive fluid resuscitation therapy. Capnography will be unable to distinguish between low $ETCO_2$ levels caused by a cardiac tamponade vs. other circulatory or metabolic issues. However, it will give the paramedic valuable trending feedback, such as an increase in $ETCO_2$ following chest decompression, helping the paramedic determine if the chosen treatment regime was successful.

Trending showcases the invaluable ability of capnography to offer continual feedback on the patient's condition to determine whether they are worsening or improving. For respiratory patients, the paramedic is confident the patient is improving when $ETCO_2$ trends lower and the slope to Phase III decreases; an increase in $ETCO_2$, or the slope to Phase III, shows a trend for the worse. In cases of circulatory and/or metabolic issues, improvement is demonstrated by a trend of increasing $ETCO_2$ levels. While many assessments offer the ability to trend, such as blood pressure, capnography is the only tool available to the paramedic that provides continual trending and does not take time to reassess once it is applied. Nonetheless, other

29

assessments are still important in painting the full clinical picture and need to be completed.

Respiratory Emergencies

There is more to interpreting capnography in respiratory patients than shark fin vs. no shark fin as the absence of a shark fin does not rule out a respiratory problem. In fact, depending on the respiratory pathology, V/Q ratio variations may be the only changes the paramedic sees in the patient's capnography. Over the next several sections the capnography of respiratory infections, asthma, COPD, CHF, PE and anxiety will be discussed in an effort to give the paramedic a broader understanding of using capnography in the context of respiratory emergencies.

Respiratory Infections

Respiratory infections usually result in no waveform shape change as most infections are not diffuse enough throughout the lungs to delay exhaled air. If a shark fin waveform is seen in a patient with a respiratory infection, the patient probably has a severe bilateral infection and/or bronchial constriction issues. Even a serious infection on one side does not usually change the waveform shape as the other side can more than compensate[1].

Variations in $ETCO_2$ levels are probably the most common capnography changes that a paramedic will see in a patient with a respiratory infection. These $ETCO_2$ changes are explained by three types of V/Q mismatches that may be present:

1. Respiratory V/Q Mismatch – obviously, a respiratory infection can interfere with gas exchange. The initial physiologic response to this is to increase RR to combat the potential hypoxia and hypercapnia. Increases in RR decrease $ETCO_2$ levels. More severe infections can cause significant respiratory distress resulting in high $ETCO_2$ levels indicating an ineffective ventilation status.
2. Circulatory V/Q Mismatch – in more severe cases, and even milder cases in the elderly, septic shock can develop. This would cause a drop in $ETCO_2$ levels secondary to compromised perfusion.

3. Simultaneous V/Q Mismatch – more than likely if the case is concerning enough to warrant a 911 call, the paramedic will encounter their patient in a simultaneous V/Q mismatch. The simultaneous V/Q mismatch of a respiratory infection would be the result of a combination of factors: an increased RR and/or septic shock would drop $ETCO_2$ while ineffective ventilations would raise $ETCO_2$ levels.

While ambiguous at times, a simultaneous V/Q mismatch can provide useful information for the paramedic. For example, consider the following scenario:

You respond to a nursing home for an 82 yoa female in respiratory distress. Upon arrival you are told by staff that the patient's symptoms have developed over the last few days. However, this morning her respiratory distress worsened. Staff denies a fever for the patient. The patient also has been complaining of dizziness and nausea. You arrive at the patient and note that she is slightly pale, in mild-moderate distress and seems to be mentating normally. You put the patient on a capnography cannula and observe a normal waveform with an RR of 28 and an $ETCO_2$ of 24. Breath sounds are diminished in all fields as the patient has a smoking history. Your partner assesses the patient's blood pressure as 108/72 with a strong regular pulse of 98 . . .

In this instance, the patient's blood pressure and pulse may or may not make the paramedic suspicious of compensated shock. However, when coupling the patient's blood pressure and pulse with the patient's capnography that shows a simultaneous V/Q mismatch, the case for compensated shock becomes more obvious. A RR of 28 is usually not enough to decrease a patient's $ETCO_2$ to 24 mmHg, alerting the paramedic to a possible circulatory/metabolic issue. In the context of this patient's clinical picture, compensated septic shock would be the first rule out. Therefore, just because a simultaneous V/Q mismatch presents some ambiguity does not mean that it is useless information. A simultaneous V/Q mismatch simply requires a full clinical picture for accurate interpretation to occur.

On a side note, while capnography can alert the paramedic to the presence of shock, it CANNOT tell the paramedic what pathology is causing the shock. For example, the capnography of septic shock and the capnography of cardiogenic shock are identical: normal waveform with low ETCO$_2$ levels. Therefore, capnography CANNOT be used to differentiate a respiratory infection from CHF. When considering giving a patient Lasix for CHF, the paramedic must first rule out a respiratory infection. Consequently, other assessments, such as lung sounds, temperature, peripheral edema, history, etc., will be needed to do this. Capnography should NEVER be the basis for Lasix administration.

In summary, capnography is very beneficial in the respiratory infection patient. It can help the paramedic identify the severity of the case, rule out the presence of a bronchial constriction issue, diagnose ineffective ventilations, trend the patient's progress throughout the call and provide continual ABC monitoring. Also, the presence of a simultaneous V/Q mismatch can help the paramedic dive deeper into the patient's pathophysiology when combined with other assessments. The pitfall of using capnography in a respiratory infection patient is that it cannot differentiate septic shock from cardiogenic shock. Therefore, other assessments should be the basis for Lasix administration, not capnography.

Asthma vs. COPD

Asthma and COPD should be considered separate disease processes because their pathophysiology and capnography are slightly different from each other. This next section will provide an explanation for this categorical change in thinking and discuss the slightly different capnography of asthma and COPD. First, consider the following scenario:

> *You respond to a 32 yoa female at a softball game complaining of difficulty breathing. Upon arrival you find the patient sitting on the grass with some of her teammates. The patient is alert and oriented with normal color and mild to moderate labored breathing. She states that about halfway through the softball game she began having an asthma attack and realized she forgot her rescue inhaler. As her condition worsened, a teammate called 911. The patient has no allergies and has a history of only asthma, for which she is prescribed two inhalers and one pill. Lung sounds reveal wheezing in all fields. Vitals are a BP of 142/80, 114 bpm strong and regular pulse, RR of 30 with an ETCO$_2$ of 33 and a shark fin type waveform with a mild slope to phase III . . .*

As previously discussed, the presence of a shark fin waveform is as diagnostic to bronchial constriction as ST elevation is to a myocardial infarction[1]. However, this patient's $ETCO_2$ is only 33, which seems counterintuitive to the CO_2 retention that a paramedic might expect to see. There are two specific considerations for this patient that the paramedic must be aware of in order to understand her capnography. First, asthma and COPD are separate pathologies and second, the capnography of asthma depends on the severity of the asthma attack while the capnography of a COPD patient is more consistent and predictable.

Asthma is better taught and discussed separately from COPD. Although research has shown a genetic pre-disposition to emphysema[12], which may explain why some patients develop emphysema without being exposed to the typical risk factors, the COPD patient is typically older and has a classic marriage between emphysema and chronic bronchitis that has developed over years of smoking and/or environmental exposure(s). Emphysema is caused by alveoli damage and chronic bronchitis is usually the result of mutated mucous production cells that create mucous uncontrollably. On the other hand, asthma is typically seen in younger patients with a primary issue of bronchial constriction that is associated with some chronic inflammation, but usually not to the degree of the COPD patient as the asthma patient's mucous cells have more normal production rates. Most notably, the typical asthma patient does not suffer from the chronic CO_2 retention often seen in COPD patients as emphysema is the primary culprit in chronic CO_2 retention and asthma patients have healthy aveoli[2]. Consequently, asthma is more of an acute pathology with minimal capnography changes outside of an exacerbation. To the contrary, COPD is a chronic condition with capnography changes that occur even without respiratory distress.

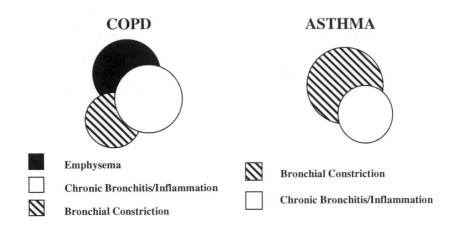

COPD

ASTHMA

- ■ Emphysema
- □ Chronic Bronchitis/Inflammation
- ▨ Bronchial Constriction

- ▨ Bronchial Constriction
- □ Chronic Bronchitis/Inflammation

The capnography of asthma is dependent on the severity of the asthma attack. Mild asthma will often result in lower than normal $ETCO_2$ levels and minimal waveform shape changes as the patient initially hyperventilates to compensate, decreasing $ETCO_2$ values. As the asthma worsens, $ETCO_2$ levels will increase and the phase III slope will steepen as a shark fin waveform begins to develop. In more severe asthma attacks, $ETCO_2$ levels rise above normal and the phase III slope slurs with a delayed phase II to create a classic shark fin appearance. The spectrum of asthma severity and its associated capnography is summarized below.

ASTHMA CAPNO	MILD	MODERATE	SEVERE
$ETCO_2$	Low	Often Normal	High
WAVEFORM	Normal	Changing	Shark Fin

The capnography of a COPD patient is different. Most COPD patients suffer from chronic CO_2 retention at rest resulting in higher than normal RR and $ETCO_2$ values and a baseline waveform that may have shark fin characteristics; all these factors quickly worsen during an exacerbation. Therefore, unless there is a compounding circulatory/metabolic issue, the capnography of a COPD exacerbation will consistently present with high $ETCO_2$ levels and usually a shark fin waveform.

All things now considered, this patient's capnography makes perfect sense as she has a primary reactive airway disease, not emphysema, and therefore will probably only suffer from CO_2 retention during a more severe asthma attack. Additionally, since her $ETCO_2$ is slightly low and her phase III slope is mild, the paramedic should interpret that the patient is having a less severe asthma attack.

In summary, while asthma patients do suffer from some degree of chronic inflammation, typically their disease process is more acute with their bronchial constriction having specific triggers. To the contrary, the typical COPD patient suffers from the chronic effects of usually emphysema and chronic bronchitis. The capnography of an asthma patient may seem counterintuitive as high $ETCO_2$ is usually present only in more severe cases. However, due to the fact that many COPD patients retain CO_2 at rest, the slightest exacerbation can quickly increase their $ETCO_2$ levels and steepen phase III of their waveform. Therefore, the paramedic should expect higher $ETCO_2$ levels and more distinguishable shark fin characteristics earlier on the spectrum of severity for COPD patients and later on the spectrum of severity for asthma patients.

CHF vs. COPD

The pathophysiology and capnography of CHF are dramatically different from COPD. Hopefully after this section the paramedic will understand why. The scenario below will serve as an illustration for this next section:

> *You respond to an 81 yoa male in an assisted living complex complaining of shortness of breath. The patient has a history of CHF and COPD and has smoked for decades. The patient appears slightly pale with mild respiratory distress and normal mentation. Lung sounds are diminished throughout all fields. However, bibasilar you think you hear what might be wheezing and/or crackles. The patient has some peripheral edema, which he describes as "normal". The patient's pulse is tachycardic, weak and thready with a blood pressure palpated at 84/P and no fever. The patient states he has recently developed a productive cough, but denies any color to his mucous. The patient's capnography shows a RR of 27 and an $ETCO_2$ of 38. His strip is shown next . . .*

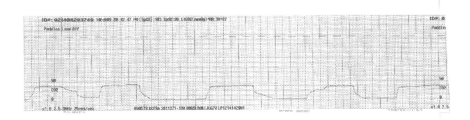

As the paramedic, you know that treating this patient aggressively with continuous Albuterol nebulizer treatments and/or using even one dose of Atrovent can worsen CHF. To the contrary, treating the patient with nitro and Lasix will not help if the primary issue is COPD; it will instead cause his condition to potentially worsen as time is wasted. While CPAP will address both etiologies, it is beneficial for the patient if the paramedic can administer the correct medications early to begin definitive treatment in the prehospital timeline. Let's take a look at this patient further and see how capnography can help the paramedic narrow the differential diagnosis, which will lead to a more clear treatment plan.

First, and this cannot be stressed enough, while capnography is an awesome tool it is still part of a bigger picture that must be completed. Capnography can help sort out the ambiguity of other assessments while other assessments can help sort out the ambiguity of capnography. Therefore, by using capnography in conjunction with the other tools available to the paramedic, the most complete clinical picture can be created.

Second, know that patients in respiratory distress with a history of both CHF and COPD will usually have components of both disease processes that are contributing to their breathing problem. The paramedic's job is to determine the primary culprit in order to administer the most beneficial treatment regime.

Now, for the capnography of CHF:

- WAVEFORM – CHF waveforms are normal in shape because CO_2 diffuses through fluid at the same rate it does through air due to CO_2's high solubility[1,2]. Even in the presence of cardiac asthma, the waveform will still be a normal shape[1]. The reason for this is that the pathology of cardiac asthma is markedly different than that of bronchial constriction. Cardiac asthma is a result of increased hydrostatic pressure in the interstitial space between the pulmonary capillary beds and the alveolar membrane. This increased pressure compresses the alveoli and terminal bronchi leading to lower airway wheezing. Hence the proverbial phrase "Not all that wheezes is asthma". Therefore, since the pathology of cardiac asthma only affects the terminal airways and is not a result of diffuse bronchial constriction, there is no waveform shape change. If a shark fin waveform is seen in a CHF patient with no history of COPD and/or asthma, the etiology is probably related to acute bronchial constriction triggered from the turbulent airflow of respiratory distress and/or a severe bilateral infection that the paramedic misinterpreted as CHF.
- $ETCO_2$ – CHF causes low $ETCO_2$ secondary to cardiogenic shock[1].
- V/Q RATIO – CHF creates a simultaneous V/Q mismatch with excessively low $ETCO_2$ secondary to cardiogenic shock and tachypnea.

Severe cases of both COPD and CHF will result in high $ETCO_2$ as ventilations become ineffective and respiratory failure looms. From a capnography perspective, waveform analysis is the best way to distinguish between etiologies in severe cases. Generally, a normal waveform rules out COPD. However, in patients with a history of both, their baseline waveform may have some shark fin characteristics. Therefore, as a general rule for patients with a history of both CHF and COPD that present with moderate to severe respiratory distress and corresponding high $ETCO_2$ levels, if the waveform is mostly normal, first rule out CHF and/or a respiratory infection; if it is mostly shark fin, first rule out COPD.

37

In summary, considering this patient's mild distress presentation, smoking and COPD history and the fact that his capnography shows a fairly normal waveform with $ETCO_2$ levels typically too low for a COPD exacerbation, his respiratory etiology is probably either caused by or has caused a circulatory issue. This line of thinking leads the paramedic to first rule out septic shock secondary to a respiratory infection and/or CHF. If this was primarily a COPD issue, the waveform would have had more impressive shark fin characteristics and the $ETCO_2$ values would be higher. Even if this patient had high $ETCO_2$, due to the waveform being mostly normal, the paramedic would probably still want to first rule out a respiratory infection and/or CHF. FYI, follow-up on this patient revealed a diagnosis of bilateral pneumonia; a great example of how the capnography of CHF and septic shock mirror each other.

Pulmonary Embolism (PE)

A PE is a block in the pulmonary circulation much like a MI is a block in the cardiac circulation. The capnography of a PE is a simultaneous V/Q mismatch secondary to decreased pulmonary perfusion and tachypnea, both contributing to excessively low $ETCO_2$ levels. The waveform is normal in a PE because there is no bronchial constriction unless the turbulent airflow of respiratory distress triggers a reactive airway syndrome. The capnography of circulatory issues, such as CHF and infection, as well as anxiety, can mimic the capnography of PE. Therefore, diagnosing PE indefinitely via capnography is impossible and requires the use of other assessments. PE is a great example of the synergistic insight achieved when capnography is coupled with other assessments. That is, the capnography of PE by itself is very ambiguous (low $ETCO_2$ and a normal waveform) as are the signs and symptoms of PE (shortness of breath with clear lung sounds that may or may not have focal chest pain, etc.). However, when both are used in conjunction with one another, they create a strong case for PE.

Anxiety

Before assuming that the cause of the patient's presentation is related to a psychiatric issue, always rule out a more serious cause of an anxiety-type presentation, such as PE. The reason for this is that the capnography of anxiety, and the presentation for that matter, is nearly identical to PE: normal waveform, high RR and low $ETCO_2$.

However, if anxiety is still the prime suspect, capnography can serve two simultaneous purposes during treatment for anxiety:

1. Coaching Visual Aid – gives the patient a numerical goal to help them control their breathing. Point out the RR value and give them incremental, quantitative RR goals to achieve as they try and slow their breathing.
2. Distraction Tool – if the paramedic can get the patient to focus on their capnography, this may distract them from what is making them upset in the first place causing their symptoms to lessen even further than just RR coaching alone.

If the paramedic is unable to increase the patient's $ETCO_2$ levels, despite a decrease in RR, and a circulatory and/or metabolic issue is ruled out, consider a PE instead of anxiety. In a PE, the $ETCO_2$ remains low despite any decreases in RR due to compromised pulmonary perfusion.

Some research has studied the use of home monitoring capnometers for patients with a long history of anxiety. These studies have shown that patients were able to increase their resting $ETCO_2$ levels by approximately 5 mmHg allowing them to recover more quickly from panic attacks. Additionally, up to 68% were "panic-attack-free" for the 12 months following the study. Capnometer home monitoring has also been useful for asthmatics who struggle with anxiety triggers helping decrease anxiety related asthma attacks.[3] Therefore, capnography is very beneficial to patients who struggle with anxiety as it is another tool to empower the patient to take control of their own breathing by giving them a visual aid while simultaneously distracting them from their situation.

Seizures

Capnography is crucial in providing insight into the ABC's of a seizure patient as capnography is not confused by motion artifact[1,4]. Without capnography, a paramedic's only assessment of a patient's airway and breathing status is "seizing" or "not seizing". With capnography, the paramedic can more specifically categorize the patient into one of three categories[5]:

1. <u>Seizing and Apneic</u> – no waveform, no RR, no $ETCO_2$ values. Be sure there is not an equipment malfunction or operator error.
2. <u>Seizing with Ineffective Ventilations</u> – most commonly represented by atypical hypoventilation (see chapter I). However, classic hypoventilation is seen as well during seizure. If tachypnea is observed with high $ETCO_2$ this is probably caused by a previous breathing pattern that caused $PaCO_2$ to rise. The high $ETCO_2$ is a cycle of effective ventilations that are working to correct hypercapnia.
3. <u>Seizing with Effective Ventilations</u> – normal waveform shape and $ETCO_2$ values.

Capnography allows the paramedic to make a more informed decision on how aggressively the patient needs to be treated and if the patient's airway and breathing status is improving or deteriorating.

Consider the following capnogram of a 10 month old female in status seizure. While this strip only gives a small snapshot of the seizure, the entire strip showed her cycling in and out of ineffective and effective breathing patterns. On the left side of the strip you see a normal waveform with an $ETCO_2$ of 66 and RR of 48. The normal waveform indicates a patent airway and the author believes that the high $ETCO_2$ is a result of the patient's previous atypical hypoventilation pattern. During her atypical hypoventilation pattern, the $PaCO_2$ built up and when she began breathing normally again, the first several breaths resulted in high $ETCO_2$. If the patient had stayed in a normal ventilation pattern long enough, her $ETCO_2$ would have most likely returned to normal. On the right side of the strip, you see atypical hypoventilation resulting in a very short waveform that then moves to apnea. This strip is a great illustration of effective ventilation, atypical hypoventilation and apnea seen in seizure:

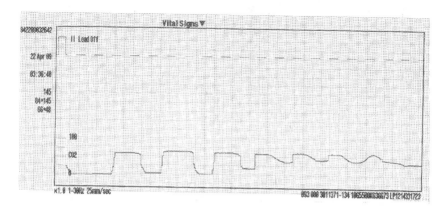

Capnography can also assist the paramedic in determining whether or not a patient has even had a seizure. This approach is somewhat ambiguous but is worth considering, particularly for those calls where a patient is found "down" and/or "altered", requiring the paramedic to wade through numerous differential diagnoses often at the mercy of poor or absent historians. Lengthy seizure activity can deplete bicarbonate reserves secondary to metabolic and respiratory acidosis from prolonged, high-intensity muscle activity coupled with a poor ventilatory status. The CO_2 circuit (see chapter II) illustrates how depleted bicarbonate decreases the ability of the body to produce CO_2, resulting in low $ETCO_2$. Therefore, if a patient has low $ETCO_2$ unexplained by ventilations or circulatory compromise, first rule out a blood sugar issue and then consider a metabolic V/Q mismatch from depleted bicarbonate secondary to a seizure. While capnography is unable to decipher what has caused low $ETCO_2$ values, the very presence of unexplained low $ETCO_2$ values in a patient who was "found down" may alert the paramedic to the possibility of a circulatory or metabolic issue more quickly than other assessments alone.

41

Non-Invasive Positive Pressure Ventilation (NIPPV)

While there is limited research on the concurrent use of capnography during NIPPV, the research that is available supports the use of capnography during NIPPV cases as it provides beneficial trending feedback on the effectiveness of treatments and the prognosis of the patient[6]. Without capnography, the noise created by NIPPV decreases the paramedic's ability to assess whether the patient is improving or worsening.

A side stream cannula under the mask is very effective and has no significant adverse leak effects on a properly positioned mask. However, a capnography device used for intubated patients on the outside of the mask should not be used as this causes CO_2 washout and inaccurate readings.[6]

Using capnography during NIPPV can also alert the paramedic to potential rebreathing that can occur during NIPPV. Rebreathing needs to be addressed, even though its effects on patient condition and prognosis have not been established in these situations.[6] There is no hard and fast rule for the paramedic to use to reverse rebreathing. Use good judgment, ensuring the breathing circuit is void of malfunctions, and remember to consider medical control for advice.

Here is a suggested sequence of how to coach a patient into NIPPV in the pre-hospital setting as well as when to apply capnography:

1. Have the patient hold the mask to their face WITHOUT applying the head harness. This will begin to get them used to the NIPPV and they will begin to realize the benefits, which is crucial to coaching them into the head harness. If the patient is too fatigued to hold the mask to their face, depending on protocol, this may be an indication that the patient needs more aggressive therapies.
2. While the patient is still holding the mask on or near their face, quickly put a capnography nasal cannula on the patient being cognizant not to disrupt their high flow oxygen therapy.
3. Next, ask the patient if they want something to help hold the mask to their face. At this point you probably could

not pry the mask out of their hands as they hopefully have realized the benefits of the NIPPV therapy, making it easier to coach them into the head harness. Once a patient is in the head harness, do NOT take the harness off to just to put capnography on. Capnography must be applied prior to the head harness.

Narcan

Capnography can also be used to titrate Narcan to RR. Administering too much Narcan too fast for a narcotic overdose can be detrimental to the patient as they wake up too quickly. This can send them into withdrawal seizures and/or make for a very messy call as they usually vomit everywhere. It can also make them very combative and violent, increasing the chance of injury to themselves and paramedics. Capnography allows the paramedic to administer small incremental doses of Narcan, just enough to raise the patient's RR. Furthermore, many narcotics will outlast Narcan and capnography can be used to determine whether the Narcan is wearing off. Additionally, capnography should be a mandatory monitoring tool for patients receiving narcotics, combined analgesia and/or procedural sedation in order to detect any problems that may arise with the patient's ABC's.

Diabetic Emergencies

Diabetic Ketoacidosis (DKA) significantly decreases $ETCO_2$ levels by depleting bicarbonate reserves secondary to prolonged metabolic acidosis. Look at the strip below of a 30 yoa male patient in DKA. This patient was found unresponsive in Kussmal's Respirations with a RR of 42 and $ETCO_2$ of 7!!

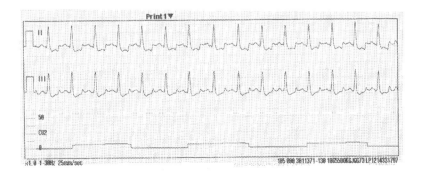

Capnography should be used in diabetic emergencies to not only constantly monitor ABC's, but also for insight into the metabolic status of the patient and the trend that treatments are having on the patient's condition. Like with circulatory issues, the paramedic would want to see an increase in $ETCO_2$ levels to indicate an improvement in the patient's metabolic status. A decline in $ETCO_2$ would indicate that the patient is worsening.

Capnography also has practical use in patients with high blood sugar as the paramedic can determine if the patient is progressing to DKA. If a patient has high blood sugar with an $ETCO_2$ lower than 30 (metabolic V/Q mismatch), the patient is probably progressing to DKA.[1,4] If a patient has high blood sugar with a normal $ETCO_2$ (normal V/Q ratio), the patient has probably not yet progressed to DKA as bicarbonate reserves are still adequate.

Malignant Hyperthermia

Malignant Hyperthermia is a rare, life threatening emergency usually caused by a patient's reactions to certain medications/drugs in an overdose or therapeutic context. While it seems to be most documented in anesthesia cases, it can also occur in the prehospital environment. The most likely scenario for a paramedic to encounter malignant hyperthermia would be in an overdose and/or an excited delirium patient that is in a hyperadrenergic state (tachycardia, increased blood pressure, tachypnia, etc.), which then leads to a severe hypermetabolic drive causing dangerously high body temperatures. Anesthesia cases and research have also documented generalized muscle rigidity as well as suggested that patients who have experienced malignant hyperthermia may have certain genetic characteristics of their skeletal muscle that contributed to the condition.[7]

Capnography can help the paramedic determine if a patient is progressing to malignant hyperthermia. After first observing the clinical signs of a hyperadrenergic state, with tachycardia often presenting first, research of humans and animals has shown that several minutes before a change in temperature can be detected, $ETCO_2$ may increase dramatically; sometimes 3-4 times the patient's previous reading.[8,9] Therefore, if a patient has clinical signs of a hyperadrenergic crisis and the paramedic notes a dramatic rise in

$ETCO_2$, consider malignant hyperthermia. This is a fatal complication and, in the opinion of the author, requires immediate physician consultation and emergent transport. Always rule out ineffective breathing as a cause of high $ETCO_2$ first. Malignant Hyperthermia is a later differential diagnosis consideration once the patient's airway and ventilation status have been confirmed to be patent and adequate.

Capnography on Circulation

Mastering the ability to use capnography to assess a patient's circulatory status through V/Q ratio determination can lead to several practical scenarios for the paramedic, such as during cardiac events, pacing, fluid resuscitation and circulatory rule outs.

Capnography can be used during an MI, or any cardiac event, to objectively assess perfusion adequacies. The "classic" MI or cardiac presentation may seem like there is no need for capnography. However, remember that capnography provides CONTINUOUS monitoring of a patient's ABC's and can trend their progress. A blood pressure, pulse, 12-lead, etc. are snapshots of one moment in time putting them at a disadvantage for trending when compared to the continuous monitoring capabilities of capnography. Also, remember that an EKG may or may not change during an MI. To the contrary, cardiac perfusion changes will affect $ETCO_2$ levels assuming circulatory compromise is the only etiology at work.

Next is the 12-lead of a 66 yoa female with sudden onset of crushing chest pain, dizziness, nausea and weakness. The patient was obtunded but alert to verbal stimuli, pale, diaphoretic with a normal respiratory effort and had the following vitals: 80/P, absent radial pulses, RR of 25 with an $ETCO_2$ of 22 and a normal waveform. 4-lead EKG showed a third degree AV block with a modified 12-lead confirming an inferior wall MI. In this case, capnography provided instant and continuous assessment of the patient's circulatory status which was crucial in complementing other assessments to complete a more in depth clinical picture.

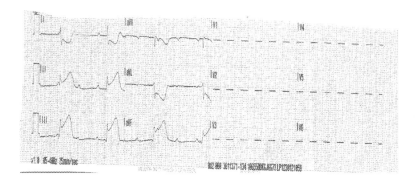

Paramedics can also use capnography to ensure that mechanical capture is obtained and maintained. Any significant increase in $ETCO_2$ levels when the paramedic initiates pacing, as well as confirmation of a pulse, indicates mechanical capture. Any unexplained drop in $ETCO_2$ levels should alert the paramedic to the possibility that mechanical capture has been lost.[1]

Capnography is reliable in low perfusion states and can be used to trend the success, or failure, of fluid resuscitation based on the change of $ETCO_2$ values.[1, 10] The paramedic optimally would like to see $ETCO_2$ trend upwards representing improvements in the patient's circulatory status. However, remember that capnography is part of a bigger picture that needs to be completed. Regular blood pressures are still crucial to ensure that the patient's blood pressure does not rise too high to avoid blowing clots that the body has created to slow bleeding.

Capnography can rule out a circulatory issue in patients with ambiguous complaints, such as dizziness, malaise, general feelings of sickness, etc., that are possibly caused by circulatory compromise. If a patient has a normal V/Q ratio, they probably do not have a circulatory/metabolic issue and the paramedic can consider a BLS track. If a patient has a V/Q mismatch, further assessment is warranted and the patient should be treated as an ALS patient.

Altitude

Altitude may decrease $ETCO_2$. This is caused by an increased RR secondary to hypoxia, which is a result of the lower partial pressure of O_2 at altitude.[11] The body compensates by increasing red blood cell production, causing the blood to become more viscous. If a person is not drinking appropriate amounts of fluids while at altitude they can become dehydrated, decreasing metabolic activity and further dropping their $ETCO_2$. Therefore, keep altitude open as an option to explain capnography changes where more common causes have already been ruled out, particularly in patients who are not acclimated and/or have a respiratory or circulatory medical history.

Many of the concepts that were presented in this chapter are more advanced and require the paramedic to first be very comfortable with the basics of capnography as well as be able to view capnography interpretation as both a science and an art. The ideas in this chapter are then a starting place for the paramedic to expand on the capabilities of capnography. Chapter IV will discuss some of the more common uses of capnography in intubated patients.

References

1. B. Krauss (personal communication, 2008 through 2009).
2. West, J.B. *Pulmonary Physiology and Pathophysiology: An Integrated, Case-Based Approach* (2nd Ed.) (6, 31 – 65). 2007. Baltimore, MD: Lippincott Williams & Wilkins.
3. Meuret A.E, Ritz, T., Dahme, T. and Roth, W.T. Therapeutic Use of Ambulatory Capnoraphy. In Gravenstein, J.S., Jaffee, M.B. and Paulus, D.A. (Ed.), *Capnography: Clinical Aspects* (129 – 135). 2004. Cambridge, U.K.: Cambridge University Press.
4. Krauss, B. Advances in the Use of Capnography for Nonintubated Patients. *Israeli Journal of Emergency Medicine*, 2008, 8: 3-15.
5. Krauss, B, Silvestri, S, and Falk, J. (2008). *Carbon dioxide monitoring (capnography)*. Retrieved October 18, 2008 from www.uptodate.com.
6. Greenway, L. Non-Invasive End-Tidal Carbon Dioxide Monitoring In Conjunction With Non-Invasive Positive Pressure Ventilation. In Gravenstein, J.S., Jaffee, M.B. and Paulus, D.A. (Ed.), *Capnography: Clinical Aspects* (137 – 141). 2004. Cambridge, U.K.: Cambridge University Press.
7. Wappler, F. (2001). Malignant Hyperthermia. *Eur. F. Anaesth.*, 18: 632-652.
8. Baudendistel, L., Goudsouzian, N., Cote, C. & Strafford, M. (1984). End-tidal CO2 monitoring: its use in the diagnosis and management of malignant hyperpyrexia. *Anaesthesia*, 39: 1000-1003.
9. De las Alas, V., Voorhees, W.P. & Geddes, L.A. (1990). End-tidal carbon dioxide concentration, carbon dioxide production, heart rate and blood pr essure as indicators of induced hyperthermia. *F. Clin. Monit.*, 6: 183-185.
10. Jin, X. et al. Decreases in Organ Blood Flows Associated with Increases in Sublingual PCO2 during Hemorrhagic Shock. *Journal of Applied Physiology*. 1998, 85: 2360-2364.
11. Schmalisch, G. Respiration at High- and Low-Pressure Environments. In Gravenstein, J.S., Jaffee, M.B. and Paulus, D.A. (Ed.), *Capnography: Clinical Aspects* (121 – 128). 2004. Cambridge, U.K.: Cambridge University Press.
12. National Institute of Health (2009). Alpha-1 Antitrypsin Deficiency. Retrieved September 3, 2009 from http://ghr.nlm.nih.gov/condition/alpha-1-antitrypsin-deficiency.

Chapter IV: Intubated Applications

While intubation has long been deemed the airway of choice in critical patients, the standard of intubation as an absolute may need to be reconsidered. Airway management should simply be to provide and/or confirm effective ventilations in all circumstances for all patients. With the successful development of supraglottic airways that now "secure" the airway at the BLS level of care, paramedic intubation may or may not be the best way to provide effective ventilations for a patient in the pre-hospital environment. Nonetheless, if intubation is deemed the best course of action for the paramedic strict guidelines should be adhered to:

> *Paramedics should be allowed to intubate only if they are using capnography as the PRIMARY means of confirming tube placement (as defined in Chapter I, "capnography" for this text assumes the congruent use of waveform and capnometer technologies unless otherwise specified). Supraglottic airways should be strongly considered after 2-3 failed intubation attempts and/or if intubation is impossible without interrupting compressions. Furthermore, following intubation, or supraglottic airway placement, paramedics must continuously monitor a patient's capnography in order to assure that the tube/supraglottic device remains patent and objective data is obtained on the patient's ABC and metabolic status. Finally, all EMS systems must establish strict quality assurance measures to ensure compliance of these guidelines.*

Confirming Tube Placement

Intubation is a difficult skill to master in the quiet and controlled operating room (OR) setting of anesthesia, let alone the loud and chaotic pre-hospital environment where intubation opportunities are limited. A study of anesthesia residents showed that an average of 57 yearly intubations were needed to achieve a 90% first attempt success rate and over 90 yearly intubations were needed for a first attempt success rate of greater than 95%[1]. A study of paramedic pre-hospital intubation showed that over 30% of patients required multiple intubation attempts, which is understandable considering the difficult situations paramedics often intubate in; on the ground in poor lightening with gunk 'n junk in the back of the throat. Overall success rates after 2-3 attempts ranged from 73%-96% with cardiac arrest having a high overall success rate of 91.8% while non cardiac arrest situations posted a meager 73.7% overall success rate. In systems with medication assisted intubation protocols, sedation showed an overall success rate of only 77.0%, but Rapid Sequence Intubation (RSI) showed the highest overall success rate of 96.3%[60].

While research shows that paramedics can indeed get the tube through the cords despite the tough prehospital intubation environment, other research taints this positive note with alarming unrecognized gut tube rates (defined as any tube outside of the trachea). In the Katz and Falk study of 2001, 108 pre-hospital patients were evaluated to determine appropriate tube placement upon arrival at the ED. The study found that up to 25% of intubated patients were delivered to the ED with a gut tube. The system where this study was conducted used capnography inconsistently[2]. Subsequent studies on other EMS systems have reported unrecognized gut tube rates of 7%-10%[3-6]. A gut tube is not a problem, unless it is unrecognized. Therefore, EMS needs to be proactively striving for an unrecognized gut tube rate of 0%. Continuous capnography monitoring is the most crucial component of reaching this goal.

If auscultation was so reliable, it would be the corner stone for tube placement used in anesthesia instead of waveform capnography. To the contrary, numerous studies have shown the unreliability of confirming tube placement through auscultation, as well as epigastric sounds, chest rise and fall and/or misting in the tube. Chest rise and fall has been observed in gut tubes and auscultation of breath sounds can be unreliable in the loud and chaotic environment of EMS[7]. In one study, auscultation of lung sounds failed to identify a gut tube 15% of the time[8]. Auscultation of gastric sounds was no more accurate when compared to breath sounds especially in thin patients. Furthermore, in one study 90% of gut tubes showed no gastric distention[7]. Another study of malpractice law suits against anesthesiologists showed that 48% of gut tubes documented "equal breath sounds"[9]. A separate study tested the ability of anesthesiologists to use breath sounds as the sole means for tube placement confirmation. Even in the quiet and controlled OR setting from the ear of a highly trained clinician, anesthesiologists were wrong 16% of the time[7]. Additionally, throughout several studies, misting in the tube has been observed in upwards of 83% of gut tubes[10]. To the contrary,

50

when waveform capnography is used properly, there is a 100% success rate in confirming tube placement both in normal and low perfusion states[6, 11-13].

After intubating a patient, observing the presence of a normal waveform (see chapter I) indicates that the tube is through the vocal cords and in the trachea. For supraglottic airways, a normal waveform indicates proper placement over the larynx. A flat line waveform or the sudden loss of a waveform usually indicates esophageal intubation/migration, but may have other causes[14]:

1. Equipment malfunction; most commonly the connection to the monitor is not tight enough and/or bodily secretions have plugged up the CO_2 sensor.
2. Try printing the strip. Many monitors reveal more from the printout than the display screen. No matter how small the waveform, if it is of normal shape, the tube is good. I have talked with paramedics that did not see any waveform on the display screen, but after printing a strip they were able to observe a very small waveform (some an $ETCO_2$ of <5!) and confirm their tube placement.
3. Prolonged down time to where cellular and alveolar death is so widespread, the body is no longer capable of any significant metabolic activity or gas exchange.
4. Poor CPR (see compressions section)
5. Complete airway obstruction below the tube
6. A "saddle block" Pulmonary Embolism (PE). A "saddle block" PE is a complete block at the bifurcation of the pulmonary artery. A saddle block PE is easily ruled out by the presence of pulses during CPR. If pulses are present, there is no saddle block PE, if they are not present, consider a complete block to the pulmonary circulation.
7. Leaking tube cuff and/or the tube has migrated to the hypopharynx; typically the waveform is an abnormal shape rather than apnea.

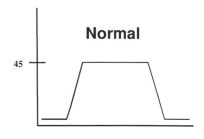

Regardless of the other possible causes of a flat line waveform besides a gut tube, paramedics should not "play the odds" while confirming or monitoring tube placement. If a flat line waveform is observed after intubation or during monitoring, ensure the equipment is attached appropriately and the CO$_2$ sensor is void of bodily secretions. The device will need to be replaced if it has become clogged; don't waste time trying to flush it out. If still no waveform is observed despite the paramedic's efforts, pull the tube or reposition the supraglottic device. It is inexcusable for paramedics to have an unrecognized gut tube because he/she thought the flat line waveform was due to less common causes: prolonged down time, low perfusion, PE, obstruction, etc. Leave your ego at the door and ALWAYS keep what is best for the patient at the center of your decisions. Would you want "the odds" played on your loved one?

Although capnography is the "gold standard" of confirming tube placement, it is unable to detect proper tube depth in a manner that is practical for the paramedic. Therefore, auscultation of equal breath sounds is still needed for verifying tube depth, but again should not be the cornerstone of tube placement verification. While one study showed a decrease of approximately 6 mmHg of ETCO$_2$ when a tube migrated right stem[15], this is not practical for EMS especially for initial intubation where there is no ETCO$_2$ baseline to compare. Therefore, use capnography first to confirm tube placement and auscultation second to confirm tube depth. Auscultation becomes a reliable "second" because what the paramedic is hearing has already been verified to be breath sounds by the confirmation of proper tube placement by capnography.

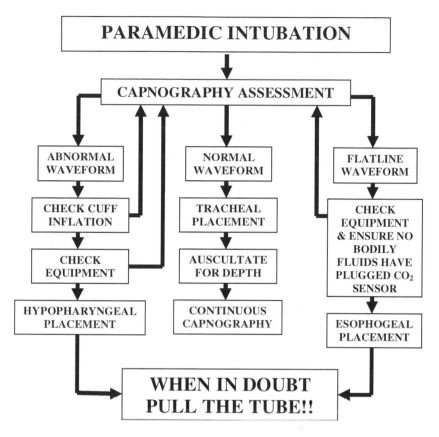

While research shows that waveform capnography and colorimetric capnography have a 100% sensitivity rate and 100% reliability rate in detecting tube placement during non-cardiac arrest situations (normal perfusion rates),[18, 55-59] waveform capnography has some significant advantages during low perfusion states where colorimetric capnography may not be sensitive enough to detect CO_2. Numerous studies have shown waveform capnography to be more sensitive than colorimetric capnography, particularly in cardiac arrest [7, 16-19]. In lower perfusion states, colorimetric capnography may not be able to detect that the tube is in the trachea when in fact the tube is properly placed; this leads to a "false negative". The author can speak to this point from personal experience where colorimetric capnography showed no color change, but waveform capnography confirmed proper tube placement. Furthermore, in the proverbial "CO_2 in the stomach" rarity, colorimetric capnography is unpredictable in how it will perform. To the contrary, waveform capnography will show an initial waveform, probably of questionable shape, and then will quickly dissipate to flat line within a handful of breaths[20-22]. Additionally, only waveform capnography is able to detect the early signs of bronchial constriction, V/Q mismatches (see chapter II), good vs. poor CPR, provide an electronic and/or hard copy record of proper tube placement, bicarbonate titrating, etc. Therefore, it is the opinion of this text that waveform capnography is superior to colorimetric capnography and should be used first with colorimetric capnography being used as a back-up technology.

Compressions, Compressions, Compressions

Numerous studies involving animals and humans have shown a reliable correlation between $ETCO_2$ and cardiac output during low perfusion states as well as during CPR[20-30]. Furthermore, these studies show that $ETCO_2$ levels change proportionally and quickly with changes in cardiac output and are accurate feedback indicators to the quality of CPR being delivered, assuming an appropriate ventilatory rate[26, 31-35]. To ensure good compressions, the paramedic should monitor $ETCO_2$ levels during CPR. If $ETCO_2$ begins to decrease, ensure that the patient is being ventilated at an appropriate rate and/or that the rescuer is not fatiguing and is providing high quality CPR. If $ETCO_2$ increases above normal, check if the patient is being under ventilated or if the patient has been resuscitated (see ROSC section). Other causes of $ETCO_2$ changes in the presence of good CPR and an appropriate ventilatory rate are PE, airway obstruction and the need for bicarbonate titration (see bicarbonate and epinephrine infusion section).

Cardiac Arrest Causation & Prognosis

Capnography has the ability to provide insight to the cause of cardiac arrest. In studies of animals and cardiac arrest patients, cardiac arrest secondary to a respiratory etiology showed initially higher $ETCO_2$ levels than cardiac arrest from a primary cardiac cause[36-38]. If a patient chokes on food that leads to cardiac arrest, the heart is still beating for several minutes before cardiac arrest occurs. Therefore, CO_2 is still being created and delivered to the lungs; hence the higher initial $ETCO_2$. To the contrary, if a patient suffers sudden cardiac death, the initial $ETCO_2$ is low as metabolic activity and CO_2 delivery to the lungs quickly collapses.

ETCO$_2$ has also been shown to be an indicator for survival rates in cardiac arrest patients. In fact, in several studies, ETCO$_2$ levels of < 10 mmHg measured after 20 minutes of paramedic intervention showed a 0% survivability rate[39-44].

Bicarbonate & Epinephrine

Research has shown temporary increases in ETCO$_2$ after the administration of Bicarbonate or Epinephrine[45]. Referring back to Chapter 1, CO$_2$ is generated through the buffering of acidic byproducts from metabolism:

$$\textbf{Acid (H}^+\textbf{)} + \textbf{Bicarbonate (HCO}_3^-\textbf{)} <=> \textbf{CO}_2 + \textbf{H}_2\textbf{O}$$

Administering bicarbonate to a patient in acidosis, such as in cardiac arrest, would cause a rise in the patient's pCO$_2$ translated to an increased ETCO$_2$, assuming that compression and ventilatory rates remain unchanged. Generally, increases in ETCO$_2$ levels from bicarbonate administration are shorter in duration than ETCO$_2$ increases seen with return of spontaneous circulation (ROSC)[46] (see ROSC section).

Bicarbonate administration should be considered if ETCO$_2$ levels begin to decrease in the presence of good CPR and an appropriate ventilatory rate. If paramedics approach bicarbonate administration from a "cookbook" approach (going through the algorithms with minimal critical thinking), potentially more harm than good can be done as extreme alkalosis is just as detrimental to a patient as extreme acidosis. Instead of giving an ambiguous "amp" of bicarbonate that usually takes the patient from acidosis to extreme alkalosis, use capnography to administer incremental, small doses of bicarbonate titrated to an appropriate ETCO$_2$ level. Additionally, if early ETCO$_2$ levels remain low despite ruling out a V/Q mismatch, an excessive ventilatory rate and/or poor CPR, consider bicarbonate administration earlier than what the cookbook calls for. Likewise, if it is 10 minutes into a cardiac arrest call and ETCO$_2$ levels are fairly normal, do not slam an amp of bicarbonate "just because". Paramedics should use capnography to determine when and how much bicarbonate is needed.

The explanation for changes in $ETCO_2$ levels during epinephrine administration is far more complex and the mechanism is not completely understood. Furthermore, unlike with bicarbonate administration, epinephrine administration has inconsistent effects on $ETCO_2$ levels. In 1992, Callaham, Barton and Matthay studied the effects of epinephrine administration on $ETCO_2$ levels. They found that $ETCO_2$ increased in 28% of the 64 cases studied, decreased in 39% and did not change in 33%[47]. Other studies have shown similar inconsistent findings[48]. Researchers have speculated several complicated physiologic theories, but no conclusions have been drawn. Therefore, for practical use for the paramedic, capnography cannot be used to guide epinephrine administration like it can with bicarbonate use.

Return of Spontaneous Circulation (ROSC)

Increases in $ETCO_2$ levels has been shown to be one of the earliest indicators of ROSC, even before a blood pressure or pulse can be measured[45, 46]. The mechanism for this is unclear, but a possible explanation is CO_2 "washout" from build-up in the blood; this is analogous to the lungs getting a "bolus" of CO_2 once the heart is able to start circulating blood on its own again[49]. As previously discussed, increases in $ETCO_2$ are also caused by bicarbonate injection and/or epinephrine administration, but the changes are short-lived where as ROSC will hopefully last much longer. If a rise in $ETCO_2$ is observed, check for a pulse to see if ROSC has occurred. If ROSC and medication administration are ruled out, consider brief "spurts" of hyperventilation to bring the patient's $ETCO_2$ back down to a more normal range. Additionally, the lack of an $ETCO_2$ increase may indicate that there is no need to check for a pulse, which can help the paramedic minimize the interruptions to compressions.

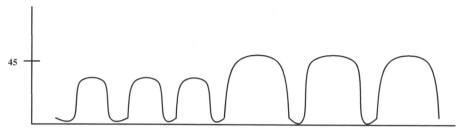

45

Possible ROSC assuming no change in CPR, ventilatory rate or recent bicarbonate or epinephrine administration

Increased Intracranial Pressure (ICP)

Capnography can help the paramedic gauge whether a patient with ICP is being ventilated at an appropriate rate as well as providing insight into their survivability. In contrast to the lungs, the brain dilates when hypoxic and constricts when well oxygenated. Hyperventilation ($ETCO_2 \leq 30$ mmHg) causes cerebral constriction resulting in decreased blood flow to the brain. To the contrary, hypoventilation ($ETCO_2 \geq 50$ mmHg) causes cerebral dilation resulting in increased blood flow to the brain[14].

Numerous research studies have not only confirmed the detriments of hyperventilation in head injury patients, but also shown that cerebral perfusion decreases almost immediately during hyperventilation, well within the time frame that a paramedic will have the patient[50-52]. On the other hand, hypoventilating a head injury patient may lead to uncontrolled hemorrhaging into the cranial vault. Therefore, a delicate balance in ICP patients is required between maintaining cerebral perfusion yet controlling cerebral hemorrhage; this dance is greatly facilitated by capnography. Be sure to follow local protocols from your medical director. However, a "permissively hypocapnic" approach to head injury patients is a good method to use. By ventilating a patient at an appropriate rate to maintain an $ETCO_2$ level of 30-35 mmHg, the paramedic can achieve the best balance possible between both cerebral perfusion maintenance and bleeding control.

Using capnography as a guide for ventilatory rates in ICP patients is supported in several research studies. In these studies, ICP patients being monitored with capnography were hyperventilated far less frequently and had increased survivability rates upon arrival at the

ED[53]. Furthermore, the capnography readings taken on these patients 20 minutes after intubation were very accurate in predicting survivability. The average $ETCO_2$ reading for survivors was 30.8 mmHg and 26.3 mmHg for those patients that died[54].

Realize that sometimes an intubated head injury patient needs little to no ventilation if they are maintaining appropriate $ETCO_2$ levels on their own. This requires an enormous amount of restraint from the paramedic. Be a paramedic with purpose. Do not bag a head injury patient simply because they are intubated. Let $ETCO_2$ govern when and how much ventilation ICP patients require.

Hopefully this chapter has shown the paramedic that confirming tube placement without capnography as the primary tool is foolish and inexcusable. Additionally, capnography can be used to guide several other decisions with intubated patients, from bicarbonate administration in cardiac arrest to identifying good vs. poor CPR and determining an appropriate ventilatory rate for head injury patients.

Like any textbook, there is no substitute for practice. If you are new to capnography, this book is a very important first step, but you have a lot of work to do before capnography can comfortably fit into your repertoire. On the other hand, if you have already been using capnography for sometime, I appreciate your open mind and the time you have invested in reading this text. Capnography needs to be a standard of care that is routinely used for assessing all types of chief complaints and presentations: respiratory, circulatory, metabolic, altered mentation, etc. Hopefully, this book has and/or will serve as the foundation for paramedics to develop a full understanding of capnography as it applies to EMS.

References

1. Konrad, C., Schüpfer, G., Wietlisbach, M. & Gerber, H. Learning manual skills in anesthesiology: is there a recommended number of cases for anesthetic procedures? *Anesth. Analg.* 1998, 86: 766-770.
2. Katz, S.H. & Falk, J.L. Misplaced endotracheal tubes by paramedics in an urban emergency medical services system. *Ann. Emerg. Med.* 2001, 37: 32-37.
3. Gausche, M, Lewis, RJ, Stratton, SJ, et al. Effect of out-of-hospital pediatric endotracheal intubation on survival and neurological outcome: a controlled clinical trial. *JAMA* 2000, 283-783.
4. Jones, JH, Murphy, MP, Dickson, RL, et al. Emergency physician-verified out-of-hospital intubation: miss rates by paramedics. *Acad. Emerg. Med.* 2004, 11: 707.
5. Jemmett, ME, Kendal, KM, Fourre, MW, Burton, JH. Unrecognized misplacement of endotracheal tubes in a mixed urban to rural emergency medical services setting. *Acad. Emerg. Med.* 2003, 10: 961.
6. Silvestri, S, Ralls, GA, Krauss, B, et al. The effectiveness of out-of-hospital use of continuous end tidal carbon dioxide monitoring on the rate of unrecognized misplaced intubation within a regional emergency medical services system. *Ann. Emerg. Med.* 2005, 45: 497.
7. Birmingham, P.K., Cheney, F.W. & Ward, R.J. Esophageal intubation: a review of detection techniques. *Anesth. Analg.* 1986, 65: 886-891.
8. Andersen, K.H. & Hald, A. Assessing the position of the tracheal tube: the reliability of different methods. *Anaesthesia.* 1989, 44: 984-985.
9. Morray, J.P., Geiduschek, J.M., Caplan, R.A., Posner, K.L., Gild, W.M. & Cheney, F.W. A comparison of pediatric and adult anesthesia closed malpractice claims. *Anesthesiology.* 1993, 78: 461-467.
10. Kelly, JJ, Eynon, CA, Kaplan, JL, et al. Use of tube condensation as an indicator of endotracheal tube placement. *Ann. Emerg. Med.* 1998, 31: 575.

11. Sayah, AJ, Peacock, WF, Overton, DT. End-tidal CO_2 measurement in the detection of esophageal intubation during cardiac arrest. *Ann. Emerg. Med.* 1990, 19: 857.
12. Silvestri, S, Heubner, M, Krauss, B, et al. Emergency department capnographic confirmation of prehospital endotracheal intubation in cardiac arrest patients – A preliminary report (abstract). *Ann. Emerg. Med.* 2005, 46: 6 (supplement).
13. Grmec, S, et al. Comparison of three different methods to confirm tracheal tube placement in emergency intubation. *Intensive Care Med.* 2002, 28: 701.
14. Krauss, B, Silvestri, S, and Falk, J. (2008). *Carbon dioxide monitoring (capnography)*. Retrieved October 18, 2008 from www.uptodate.com.
15. Gandhi, S.K., Munshi, C.A., Coon, R. & Bardeen-Henschel, A. Capnography for detectin of endobronchial migration of an endotracheal tube. *F. Clin. Monit.* 1991, 7: 35-38.
16. Hayden, S.R., Sciammarella, J., Viccelo, P., Thode, H. & Delagi, R. Colorimetric end-tidal CO_2 detection for verification of endotracheal tube placement in out-of-hospital cardiac arrest. *Acad. Emerg. Med.* 1995, 2: 499-502.
17. MacLeod, B.A., Heller, M.B., Gerard, J., Yealy, D.M. & Menegazzi, J.J. Verification of endotracheal tube placement with colorimetric end-tidal CO_2 detection. *Ann. Emerg. Med.* 1991, 20: 267-270.
18. Ornato, J.P., Shipley, J.B., Racht, E.M., Slovis, C.M., Wrenn, K.D., Pepe, P.E., Almeida, S.L., Ginger, V.F. & Fotre, T.V. Multicenter study of a portable, hand-size, colorimetric end-tidal carbon dioxide detection device. *Ann. Emerg. Med.* 1992, 21: 518-523.
19. Bozeman, WP, Hexter, D, Liang, HK, Kelen, GD. Esophageal detector device versus detection of end-tidal carbon dioxide level in emergency intubation. *Ann. Emerg. Med.* 1996, 27: 595.
20. Isserles, A.A. & Breen, P.H. Can changes in end-tidal PCO2 measure changes in cardiac output? *Anesth. Analog.* 1991, 73: 808-814.
21. Idreis, A.H., Staples, E.D., O'Brien, D.J., et al. End-tidal carbon dioxide during extremely low cardiac output. *Ann. Emerg. Med.* 1994, 23: 568-572.

22. Jin, X., Weil, M.H., Tang, W., et al. End-tidal carbon dioxide as a noninvasive indicator of cardiac index during circulatory shock. *Crit. Care Med.* 2000, 28: 2415-2419.

23. Trevino, R.P., Bisera, J., Weil, M.H., Rackow, E.C. & Grundler, W.G. End-tidal CO_2 as a guide to successful cardiopulmonary resuscitation: a preliminary report. *Crit. Care Med.* 1985, 13: 910-911.

24. Weil, M.H., Bisera, J., Trevino, R.P. & Rackow, E.C. Cardiac output and end-tidal carbon dioxide. *Crit. CareMed.* 1985, 13: 907-909.

25. Grundler, W., Weil, M.H. & Rackow, E.C. Arteriovenous carbon dioxide and pH gradients during cardiac arrest. *Circulation.* 1986, 74: 1071-1074.

26. Gudipati, C.V., Weil, M.H., Bisera, J., Deshmukh, H.G. & Rackow, E.C. Expired carbon dioxide: a noninvasive monitor of cardiopulmonary resuscitation. *Circulation.* 1988, 77: 234-239.

27. Falk, J.L., Rackow, E.C. & Weil, M.H. End-tidal carbon dioxide concentration during cardiopulmonary resuscitation. *New. Engl. F. Med.* 1988, 318: 607-611.

28. Ornato, J.P., Garnett, A.R. & Glauser, F.L. Relationship between cardiac output and the end-tidal carbon dioxide tension. *Ann. Emerg. Med.* 1990, 19: 1104-1106.

29. Shibutani, K., Muraoka, M., Shirasaki, S., Kubbal, K., Sanchala, V.T. & Gupte, P. Do changes in end-tidal PCO_2 quantitatively reflect changes in cardiac output? *Anesth. Analog.* 1994, 79: 829-833.

30. Blumenthal, S.R. & Voorhees, W.D. The relationship of carbon dioxide excretion during cardiopulmonary resuscitation to regional blood flow and survival. *Resuscitation.* 1997b, 35: 135-143.

31. Garnett, A.R., Ornato, J.P., Gonzalez, E.R. & Johnson, E.B. End-tidal carbon dioxide monitoring during cardiopulmonary resuscitation. *F. Am. Assoc.* 1987, 257: 512-515.

32. Lepilin, M.G., Vasilyev, A.V., Bildinov, O.A. & Rostovtseva, N.A. End-tidal carbon dioxide as a noninvasive monitor of circulatory status during cardiopulmonary resuscitation: a preliminary clinical study. *Crit. Care Med.* 1987, 15: 958-959.

33. Ward, K.R., Menegazzi, J.J., Zelenak, R.R., Sullivan, R.J. & McSwain, Jr., N.E. A comparison of chest compressions between mechanical and manual CPR by monitoring end-tidal

PCO$_2$ during human cardiac arrest. *Ann. Emerg. Med.* 1993, 22: 669-674.

34. Blumenthal, S.R. & Voorhees, W.D. The relationship between airway carbon dioxide excretion and cardiac output during cardiopulmonary resuscitation. *Resuscitation.* 1997a, 34: 263-270.
35. Kalenda, Z. The capnogram as a guide to the efficacy of cardiac massage. *Resuscitation.* 1978, 6: 259-263.
36. Bhende, M.S., Karasic, D.G., Karasic, R.B. End-tidal carbon dioxide changes during cardiopulmonary resuscitation after experimental asphyxial cardiac arrest. *Am. J. Emerg. Med.*, 1996. 14:349.
37. Berg, R.A., Henry, C., Otto, C.W., et al. Initial end-tidal CO$_2$ is markedly elevated during cardiopulmonary resuscitation after asphyxial cardiac arrest. *Pediatr. Emerg. Care*, 1996. 12: 245.
38. Grmec, S., Lah, K., Tusek-Bunc, K. Difference in end-tidal CO$_2$ between asphyxia cardiac arrest and ventricular fibrillation/pulseless ventricular tachycardia cardiac arrest in the prehospital setting. *Crit. Care*, 2003. 7: R139.
39. Sanders, A.B., Kern, K.B., Otto, C.W., et al. End-tidal carbon dioxide monitoring during cardiopulmonary resuscitation. A prognostic indicator for survival. *JAMA*, 1989. 262: 1347.
40. Levin, R.L., Wayne, M.A., Miller, C.C. End-tidal carbon dioxide and outcome of out-of-hospital cardiac arrest. *N. Engl. J. Med.*, 1997. 337: 301.
41. Wayne, M.A., Levine, R.L., Miller, C.C. Use of end-tidal carbon dioxide to predict outcome in prehospital cardiac arrest. *Ann. Emerg. Med.*, 1995. 25: 762.
42. Grmec, S, Klemen, P. Does the end-tidal carbon dioxide (etCO2) concentration have prognostic value during out-of-hospital cardiac arrest. *Eur. J. Emerg. Med.*, 2001. 8: 263.
43. Sanders, A.B., Ewy, G.A., Bragg, S., et al. Expired PCO2 as a prognostic indicator of successful resuscitation from cardiac arrest. *Ann. Emerg. Med.*, 1985. 14: 948.
44. Asplin, B.R., White, R.D., Prognostic value of end-tidal carbon dioxide pressures during out-of-hospital cardiac arrest. *Ann. Emerg. Med.* 1995. 25: 756.
45. Garnett, A.R., Ornato, J.P., Gonzalez, E.R. & Johnson, E.B. End-tidal carbon dioxide monitoring during cardiopulmonary resuscitation. *F. Am. Assoc.* 1987, 257: 512-515.

46. Falk, J.L., Rackow, E.C. & Weil, M.H. End-tidal carbon dioxide concentration during cardiopulmonary resuscitation. *New Engl. F. Med.* 1988, 318: 607-611.
47. Callaham, M., Barton, C. & Matthay, M. Effect of epinephrine on the ability of end-tidal carbon dioxide readings to predict initial resuscitation from cardiac arrest. *Crit. Care Med.* 1992, 20: 337-343.
48. Cantineau, J.P., Merckx, P., Lambert, Y., Sorkine, M., Bertrand, C. & Duvaldestin, P. Effect of epinephrine on end-tidal carbon dioxide pressure during prehospital cardiopulmonary resuscitation. *Am. F. Emerg. Med.* 1994, 12: 267-270.
49. B. Krauss (personal communication, 2008 through 2009).
50. Bao, Y., Jiang, J., Zhu, C., Lu, Y., Cai, R. & Ma, C. Effect of hyperventilation on brain tissue oxygen pressure, carbon dioxide pressure, pH value and intracranial pressure during intracranial hypertension in pigs. *Chin. F. Traumatol.* 2000, 3: 210-213.
51. Marion, D.W., Puccio, A., Wisniewski, S.R., Kochanek, P., Dixon, C.E., Bullian, L. & Carlier, P. Effect of hyperventilation on extracellular concentrations of glutamate, lactate, pyruvate, and local cerebral blood flow in patients with severe traumatic brain injury. *Crit. Care Med.* 2002, 30: 2619-2625.
52. Sarrafzadeh, A.S., Sakowitz, O.W., Callsen, T.A., Lanksch, W.R. & Unterberg, A.W. Detection of secondary insults by brain tissue PO_2 and bedside microdialysis in severe head injury. *Acta. Neurochir.* 2002, Suppl. 81: 319-321.
53. Helm, M., Schuster, R., Hauke, J., Lampl, L. Tight control of prehospital ventilation by capnography in major trauma victimes. *Br. J. Anaesth.*, 2003, 90: 327.
54. Deakin, C.D., Sado, D.M., Coats, T.J., Davies, G. Prehospital end-tidal carbon dioxide concentration and outcome in major trauma. *J. Trauma.*, 2004, 57: 65.
55. Goldberg, J.S., Rawle, P.R., Zehnder, J.L., Sladen, R.N. Colorimetric end-tidal carbon dioxide monitoring for tracheal intubation. *Anesth. Analg.*, 1990, 70: 191.
56. Knapp, S. Kofler, J., Stoiser, B. et. al. The assessment of four different methods to verify tracheal tube placement in the critical care setting. *Anesth. Analg.*, 1999, 88: 766.

57. MacLeod, B.A., Heller, M.B., Gerard, J. et. al. Verification of endotracheal tube placement with colorimetric end-tidal CO_2 detector. *Ann. Emerg. Med.*, 1991, 20: 267.
58. Vukmir, R.B., Heller, M.B., Stein, K.L. Confirmation of endotracheal tube placement: A miniaturized infrared qualitative CO_2 detector. *Ann. Emerg. Med.*, 1991, 20: 726.
59. Grmec, S., Mally, S. Prehospital determination of tracheal tube placement in severe head injury. *Emerg. Med. J.*, 2004, 21: 518.
60. Wang, H.E., Yealy, D.M. How Many Attempts Are Required to Accomplish Out-of-Hospital Endotracheal Intubation? *Academic Emerg. Med.*, 2006, 13: 372-377.

Capnography Cliff Notes

This section attempts to summarize the important concepts of the book. If you are less familiar with capnography, it is recommended that you read the book in its entirety before reading this section. However, if you have already been through the text and/or are already familiar with capnography, this section can serve as a quick review and/or help identify concepts that you want to further explore. Once you find a specific topic here, you can refer back to that section of the book for a more in depth explanation.

The Basics

- Carbon Dioxide (CO_2) is the "smoke" of metabolism, a concept first documented by the Greeks. The Greek work for smoke is "Capnos", hence the origin of the word "Capnography".
- Capnography uses infrared technology to measure CO_2 in exhaled air. The findings are displayed via waveform, a color change and/or numerical values, which often also include the patient's respiratory rate (RR).
- Capnography is a powerful diagnostic test, but absolutely must be interpreted in the clinical context of the patient. Otherwise, inaccurate conclusions are inevitable.
- Capnography directly measures ventilation, but is a good tool for assessing a patient's circulatory/metabolic status.
- Pulse oximetry directly measures hemoglobin saturation and indirectly indicates oxygen saturation and can give false readings, such as in carbon monoxide poisoning. Therefore, while capnography is a stand alone technology, pulse oximetry is not and should be used in conjunction with capnography and/or other assessments.
- CO_2 is created by buffering the acidic byproducts of metabolism where acid combines with bicarbonate to create CO_2 and water.
- End Tidal Carbon Dioxide ($ETCO_2$) is the term used for the amount of CO_2 detected in exhaled air and is measured in mmHg.

- Waveform capnography is the most common display of capnography used in EMS. It provides a numerical value for $ETCO_2$ and RR as well as a waveform.
- There are 2 categories of waveforms: physiologic and artifact. As the name implies, physiologic waveforms are a direct result of patient physiology while artifact waveforms are not.

A Systematic Approach

- To implement capnography on a routine basis, a systematic approach can be beneficial to the paramedic.
- To ensure that capnography is interpreted in the clinical picture of the patient a 3 step process is used: initial impression, waveform analysis and V/Q ratio assessment. As the paramedic becomes more familiar with capnography, he/she can make this process unique to their style of medicine.
- First, develop an initial impression. This is done by observing the patient's color, mentation and respiratory effort and providing immediate BLS interventions that are necessary, such as high flow oxygen, before moving onto capnography. The initial impression is the foundation of painting the clinical picture of the patient and is dynamic and often changing as more information is gathered.
- Next, apply capnography and observe the patient's waveform and decide what is categorically revealed about the patient, interpreting the waveform in the context of the initial impression, chief complaint, etc.
- Finally, determine the patient's V/Q ratio. While complicated, the V/Q ratio is the nuts and bolts of capnography and failure to understand this concept denies the paramedic the ability to utilize capnography to its fullest potential.
- Understanding the CO_2 circuit is crucial in order to comprehend how a V/Q assessment is obtained through capnography.
- The V/Q ratio compares the volume of air being ventilated with the amount of blood being delivered to the lungs via the pulmonary circulation. A V/Q mismatch occurs when this delicate "tug-of-war" between ventilation and pulmonary perfusion "seesaws" out of balance.

- Capnography can only qualitatively, not quantitatively, assess the patient's V/Q ratio putting the patient's V/Q ratio into 1 of 4 categories: Normal, Respiratory Mismatch, Circulatory/Metabolic Mismatch, or Simultaneous Mismatch.

Non-Intubated Applications

- To use capnography in non-intubated patients in EMS, a side stream cannula is utilized.
- Use capnography to trend a patient's improvements and/or progression for the worse.
- A respiratory emergency is probably the most common use for capnography by paramedics. Scenarios and applications of capnography in this context are respiratory infections, asthma, COPD, CHF, PE and anxiety.
- Know that capnography alone cannot determine whether Lasix is appropriate. Other assessments MUST be used.
- Capnography can be used during seizures to more specifically assess a patient's respiratory status. Additionally, capnography can be coupled with other assessments to see if a patient has even had a seizure. This approach is somewhat ambiguous but is worth considering, particularly for those calls where a patient is found "down" and/or "altered" requiring the paramedic to wade through numerous differential diagnoses often at the mercy of poor, or absent, historians.
- Use capnography during Non-Invasive Positive Pressure Ventilation (NIPPV) therapies, such as Continuous Positive Airway Pressure (CPAP), to trend the patient's progress and ensure that rebreathing does not occur.
- Capnography can be used to titrate Narcan and is a monitoring must when administering narcotics and/or combined analgesia to a patient.
- Diabetic patients presenting with high blood sugar benefit from capnography as the paramedic can determine if the patient has progressed to Diabetic Ketoacidosis (DKA), or if bicarbonate levels are still adequate.
- Changes in a patient's capnography can be an early indicator for malignant hyperthermia.

- Once the paramedic understands the CO_2 circuit and V/Q ratio capabilities of capnography, there are several uses for capnography on circulatory assessment: cardiac events, confirming and monitoring mechanical capture, trending fluid resuscitation efforts and triaging ambiguous patient complaints.
- If applicable, remember altitude as a differential diagnosis to changes in a patient's capnography; this is particularly important in patients who have recently traveled to altitude and may have medical problems that predispose them to difficulties with acclimation.

Intubated Applications

- Intubation is arguably the most common application of capnography.
- The research is overwhelming and undeniable: paramedics who do not use waveform capnography as the PRIMARY means for confirming proper tube placement needlessly put their patient's at risk for an inexcusable gut tube.
- Paramedics who use waveform capnography correctly have a 100% success rate of confirming tube placement.
- Auscultation of breath sounds in anesthesia, let alone the loud and chaotic environment of EMS, has been shown in numerous studies to be unreliable in determining tube placement.
- Other assessments for confirming tube placement, such as epigastric sounds, chest rise and fall, misting in the tube, etc., have also been shown to be unreliable.
- Auscultation is still needed to confirm tube depth, but only after waveform capnography has confirmed that what the paramedic is hearing is in fact breath sounds. If auscultation were so reliable, it would be the corner stone used in anesthesia instead of waveform capnography.
- Waveform capnography is a far superior technology to colorimetric capnography.
- Use capnography to determine the quality of compressions being delivered during CPR.
- Capnography can help differentiate the cause of cardiac arrest: respiratory versus sudden cardiac death. Also, capnography

can be used as a reliable indicator for prognosis in cardiac arrest.

- Use capnography to determine when and how much bicarbonate to infuse. Do not be a cook book medic, slamming amps of bicarbonate robotically without thought. Use capnography and think!

- Capnography is one of the earliest indicators of the Return of Spontaneous Circulation (ROSC), before a blood pressure or a pulse can be assessed.

- Use capnography to ensure that intubated patients with increased intracranial pressure (ICP) are ventilated at an appropriate rate. This is done using a permissively hypocapnic approach. Some ICP patients will require intubation only for securing the airway and will not need to be ventilated.

From simple ABC and metabolic monitoring to V/Q mismatch determination and medication administration during cardiac arrest, capnography is a powerful diagnostic tool, arguably the best that paramedics carry. Capnography can provide continual and simultaneous monitoring of the patient's airway, breathing and metabolic status whereas other assessments, while still important, are more limited.

Like any textbook, there is no substitute for practice. If you are new to capnography, this book is a very important first step, but you have a lot of work to do before capnography can comfortably fit into your repertoire. On the other hand, if you have already been using capnography for sometime, I appreciate your open mind and the time you have invested in reading this text. Capnography needs to be a standard of care that is routinely used for assessing all types of chief complaints and presentations: respiratory, circulatory, metabolic, altered mentation, etc. Hopefully, this book has and/or will serve as the foundation for all paramedics to develop a full understanding of capnography as it applies to EMS.